Critical
Thinking Skills for your
Education
Degree

Critical Study Skills for Education Students

Our new series of study skills texts for teacher training and other education professional students has four key titles to help you succeed in your degree:

Studying for your Education Degree

Academic Writing and Referencing for your Education Degree

Critical Thinking Skills for your Education Degree

Communication Skills for your Education Degree

Register with **Critical Publishing** to:

- be the first to know about forthcoming education titles;
- find out more about our new series;
- sign up for our regular newsletter for special offers, discount codes and more.

Visit our website at: 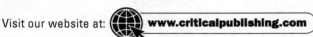 **www.criticalpublishing.com**

Our titles are also available in a range of electronic formats. To order please go to our website www.criticalpublishing.com or contact our distributor NBN International by telephoning 01752 202301 or emailing orders@nbninternational.com.

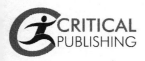

Critical
Thinking Skills for your
Education
Degree

CRITICAL
STUDY SKILLS

ANE BOTTOMLEY, KULWINDER MAUDE, STEVEN PRYJMACHUK AND DAVID WAUGH

First published in 2019 by Critical Publishing Ltd

The authors have made every effort to ensure the accuracy of information contained in this publication, but assume no responsibility for any errors, inaccuracies, inconsistencies and omissions. Likewise every effort has been made to contact copyright holders. If any copyright material has been reproduced unwittingly and without permission the Publisher will gladly receive information enabling them to rectify any error or omission in subsequent editions.

British Library Cataloguing in Publication Data
A CIP record for this book is available from the British Library

ISBN: 978-1-912508-57-0

This book is also available in the following e-book formats:

MOBI: 978-1-912508-58-7
EPUB: 978-1-912508-59-4
Adobe e-book reader: 978-1-912508-60-0

The rights of Jane Bottomley, Kulwinder Maude, Steven Pryjmachuk and David Waugh to be identified as the Authors of this work have been asserted by them in accordance with the Copyright, Design and Patents Act 1988.

Text and cover design by Out of House Limited
Project Management by Newgen Publishing UK
Printed and bound in Great Britain by 4edge, Essex

Critical Publishing
3 Connaught Road
St Albans
AL3 5RX

www.criticalpublishing.com

Paper from responsible sources

Contents

Acknowledgements

We would like to thank the many university students who have inspired us to write these books. Special thanks are due to Anita Gill. Particular appreciation goes to students at Kingston University and Durham University. Special thanks are due to Simon Parry, Senior Lecturer at Kingston University, and Sohang Tang, PGCE secondary maths student at Kingston University, for giving us permission to use their reflective writing essays as samples for this book, and to other students who gave their permission for their work to be used anonymously. Many thanks to Vin Wynne of the National Education Union for providing case studies. Thanks also to Julia Morris at Critical Publishing for her support and editorial expertise.

Jane Bottomley, Kulwinder Maude, Steven Pryjmachuk and David Waugh

The Publishers would also like to express their grateful thanks for permission to use the following text extracts within this book:

- Brundrett, M (2013) The Importance of Teachers, Teaching and School Leaders: The 'Silver Thread' of the Reform Agenda for English Schools. *Education 3-13: International Journal of Primary, Elementary and Early Years Education*, 41(5), 459–61.
- Darnell, C, Solitya, J and Walla, H (2017) Decoding the Phonics Screening Check. *British Educational Research Journal*, 43(3), 505–27.
- Glazzard, J (2017) Assessing Reading Development through Systematic Synthetic Phonics. *English in Education*, 51(1), 44–57.

Meet the authors

Jane Bottomley

is a freelance writer, teacher and educational consultant. She is a Senior Fellow of the Higher Education Academy and a Senior Fellow of the BALEAP, the global forum for English for Academic Purposes practitioners. She has helped students from a wide range of disciplines to improve their academic skills and achieve their study goals, including 14 years as a Senior Language Tutor at the University of Manchester. Jane is the editor of the *Critical Study Skills* series, which covers nursing, education and social work.

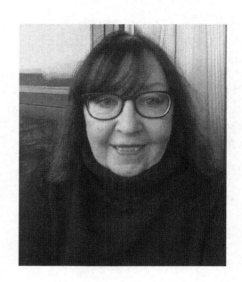

Kulwinder Maude

is a Senior Lecturer at Kingston University, London. She has over 20 years of experience working in different sectors of education, including extensive experience of teaching and learning in primary schools (England and India) as well as UK higher education. She teaches English on undergraduate and postgraduate Initial Teacher Education (ITE) programmes along with teaching a Masters-level module on reflective teaching. She has written articles and chapters on many aspects of primary English for ITE and primary practitioners.

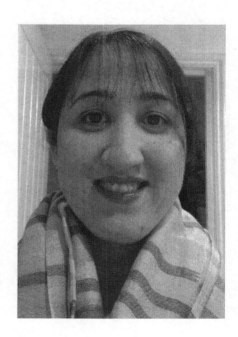

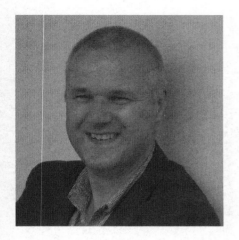

Steven Pryjmachuk

is Professor of Mental Health Nursing Education in the School of Health Sciences' Division of Nursing, Midwifery and Social Work at the University of Manchester and a Senior Fellow of the Higher Education Academy. His teaching, clinical and research work has centred largely on supporting and facilitating individuals – be they students, patients or colleagues – to develop, learn or care independently.

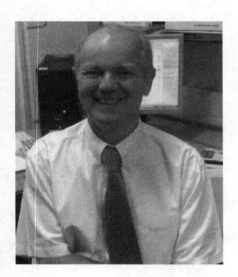

David Waugh

is Associate Professor of Education at Durham University. He has written more than 50 books on education and has taught in four schools, as well as teaching undergraduates and postgraduates and providing professional development for teachers. He has worked in universities for 29 years and still regularly teaches in schools using the children's novels he writes as a stimulus for reading, writing and discussion.

Introduction

Critical Thinking Skills is the third book in the *Critical Study Skills for Education* series. This series supports student teachers and education professionals as they embark on their undergraduate degree programme. It is aimed at all student teachers, including those who have come to university straight from A levels, and those who have travelled a different route, perhaps returning to education after working and/or raising a family. The books will be of use both to students from the UK and to international students who are preparing to study in a new culture – and perhaps in a second language. The books also include guidance for students with specific learning requirements.

Critical Thinking Skills aims to remove some of the 'mystique' which often surrounds critical thinking – students sometimes hear that they are 'not critical' enough but may struggle to understand just what this means in practical terms. This book guides you towards an understanding of critical thinking and its role in academic and professional life, with plain-English explanations and practical examples provided throughout. It discusses the importance of questioning what you see and hear, and equips you with a range of analytical and evaluative tools. It places reflective practice at the heart of critical thinking and provides language tools which can help you express your reflections more precisely. It provides strategies to help you read and write critically, using the research and writing process to discover and develop your own voice, an essential part of being a critical scholar.

Between them, the authors have many years' experience of both school teaching and education, and academic study skills. All the information, text extracts and activities in the book have a clear education focus and are often directly linked to the Teachers' Standards (DfE, 2011).

The many activities in the book include **tasks**, **reflections**, **top tips**, and **case studies**. There are also **advanced skills** sections which highlight particular knowledge and skills that you will need towards the end of your degree programme – or perhaps if you go on to postgraduate study. The activities in the book often require you to work things out and discover things for yourself, a learning technique which is commonly used in universities. For many activities, there is no right or wrong answer – they might simply require you to reflect on your experience or situations you are likely to encounter at university; for tasks which require a particular response, there is an answer key at the back of the book.

These special features throughout the book are clearly signalled by icons to help you recognise them:

 Learning outcomes;

 Quick quiz or example exam questions/assessment tasks;

 Reflection (a reflective task or activity);

 Case studies;

 Top tips;

Checklist;

 Advanced skills information;

 Answer provided at the back of the book.

Students with limited experience of academic life in the UK will find it helpful to work through the book systematically; more experienced students may wish to 'dip in and out' of the book. Whichever approach you adopt, handy **cross references** signalled in the margins will help you quickly find the information that you need to focus on or revisit.

There are two **Appendices** (Academic levels at university; Verb forms in English) at the back of the book, which you can consult as you work through the text.

We hope that this book will help you to develop as a critical education student, and to become a confident member of your academic community.

A note on terminology

In the context of this book, the term 'education' should be used to include 'teaching, teacher training and the allied education professionals' wherever this is not explicitly stated.

Chapter 1
The foundations of critical thinking

Learning outcomes

After reading this chapter you will:

- better understand what is meant by 'critical thinking';

- better understand the relevance and importance of critical thinking in the theory and practice of education;

- have begun to learn how to apply critical thinking to your studies and to your education practice.

There are many books and courses in schools, colleges and universities entitled 'Critical Thinking' (like this book!), a fact which reflects its importance in education, particularly in universities. However, critical thinking is not a discrete study topic like those in other books and modules you may encounter (for example, 'English, maths and science knowledge and understanding in primary education' or 'Pedagogy and school experience'); critical thinking is actually threaded through every aspect of your studies and your practice.

This chapter helps you begin to trace and understand this thread. It explores important aspects of critical thinking in academic study and in educational practice, in particular, the importance of objectively questioning the information and ideas you encounter. Chapter 2 explores reflective practice, which is closely related to critical thinking and is a key aspect of teaching. Chapters 3 and 4 cover how to *apply* critical thinking skills in your academic reading and writing.

Of course, it is not possible to think critically about an education topic if you are not grounded in the *knowledge* of your discipline, and all the guidance and tasks in this book will be rooted in your developing knowledge of education theory and practice.

CROSS REFERENCE

Chapter 2, Reflective practice

CROSS REFERENCE

Chapter 3, Critical reading

CROSS REFERENCE

Chapter 4, Critical writing

Reflection

1) What do you understand by the term 'critical thinking'?

2) Why do you think critical thinking, as you understand it, is so important across education and professional practice?

3) Which parts of the Teachers' Standards make reference to critical thinking?

4) Have you ever received feedback from a teacher or lecturer which said you had not been critical enough? Did you understand what you had done wrong?

5) Have you felt that something you recently read or heard was lacking in critical thinking? Why?

6) In what ways do you think you can demonstrate criticality in your studies and/or your teaching practice?

Asking the right questions

A good place to start with critical thinking is with the idea of asking questions in order to get to the truth. This idea can be traced back to the ancient Greek philosopher Socrates, who is said to have laid down the roots of western philosophy by questioning everything around him, and by demonstrating time and again that seemingly knowledgeable people, himself included, often didn't really know what they thought they knew!

> An example [of Socrates' questioning approach] was his conversation with Euthydemus. Socrates asked him whether being deceitful counted as being immoral. Of course it does, Euthydemus replied. He thought that was obvious. But what, Socrates asked, if your friend is feeling very low and might kill himself, and you steal his knife? Isn't that a deceitful act? Of course it is. But isn't it moral rather than immoral to do that? It's a good thing, not a bad one – despite being a deceitful act.
>
> (Warburton, 2012, p 2)

Socrates' thinking may seem like common sense: most of us can think of examples of 'deceit' – the telling of 'white lies', for instance – which are intended to help rather than harm people. But the important point is that Socrates was questioning received wisdom and relying solely on reasoned argument to arrive at the truth. The use of questioning and reasoned argument is central to academic and professional practice. This means, in essence, *not believing things merely because someone important says they are true*, and making sure your own beliefs are constructed around sound reasoning and credible evidence.

Knowledge and understanding in educational theory and practice are developing all the time. This inevitably means that sometimes there are instances of received wisdom which turn out to be wrong. This may be because not enough was known about a particular thing at a given time, or it may be that people did not ask enough questions – or at least the *right* questions.

Task

Exploring changes in thinking 1

Look at the case studies below (the first one is a very general example relating to consumerism and health care, but of interest in terms of the types of concerns parents have regarding their children's well being; the second relates to an issue in education) and answer these questions:

1) What was the current knowledge or 'received wisdom' in each case?

2) How was this challenged?

3) What, if anything, do you think should happen now?

Case studies

The Nappy Science Gang

When shopping for washing powder in any UK supermarket, we are faced with the choice of biological or non-biological detergents. Many of us may not be sure of the difference between them, but the information generally available to consumers suggests that biological detergents are more powerful and better at removing dirt and stains because they contain enzymes (substances that speed up chemical reactions, in relation to cleaning in this case). Ideal for very dirty items like nappies, you might think. However, NHS advice, as reported through the *NHS Choices* website, has long been to wash babies' nappies in *non-biological* detergent, which seems to reflect the general belief among the UK population that biological detergents irritate the skin. Nappy manufacturers and other organisations traditionally aligned themselves with NHS advice. However, in 2015, *The Guardian* reported that the *Nappy Science Gang*, a citizens' science project supported by the *Wellcome Trust* and the *Royal Society of Chemistry*, had been questioning the NHS advice on detergent use. This group of parents cited studies which appeared to show that biological detergents were no more likely to cause skin irritation than non-biological detergents, with no connection being found between enzymes and skin complaints. They also pointed to the fact that this 'myth' of enzyme irritation appeared not to exist in other countries, where, in fact, it can be pretty difficult to find non-biological detergents. The *Nappy Science Gang* asked *NHS Choices* to investigate the evidence base for the advice they were issuing on their website. After consulting the literature and experts in the field, the NHS reported that they would be changing the advice given on their website. So, as reported in *The Guardian*, thanks to 'a bunch of volunteer mums who wouldn't stop asking questions' (Collins, 2015), and the readiness of the NHS to listen, advice on the *NHS Choices* website now reads: 'There's no evidence that using washing powders with enzymes (bio powders) or fabric conditioners will irritate your baby's skin.'

Phonics test results are a credit to the government (or are they?)

When a new Conservative government came into office in 2010, they placed a great deal of emphasis on the importance of teaching systematic synthetic phonics (SSP).Central to this was the introduction of phonics screening tests in 2012. A great deal of teaching centred on preparing children for these tests, and the outcomes were very positive.

An article written in *The Guardian* by an academic from Durham University (Waugh, 2014) acknowledged that improved screening test results were very welcome and a good example of how consistent educational policies can bring benefits to children. However, he also noted that the policies he was citing in fact reflected credit on the previous Labour government (1997–2010), who were the first government to introduce a strong emphasis on the teaching of systematic synthetic phonics. Waugh was questioning claims or assumptions in order to establish the true source of a successful policy.

In another important development, the review of literacy teaching by Sir Jim Rose, again commissioned by the Labour government in 2006, placed great emphasis upon phonics being taught in the context of a broad, rich language curriculum, with lots of experience of good-quality literature. The subsequent Conservative government introduced a new national curriculum that stresses the importance of sharing literature with children. However, it is yet to be seen whether this will inculcate those young readers who have acquired basic phonics skills with a real desire to read for pleasure and purpose (Waugh, 2014). Policy makers and teachers will need to view developments in this area with a critical, questioning eye.

The two case studies you have analysed are good examples of how experts question the existing public discourse or need to change their thinking when confronted with new evidence. There are many other areas of public life and education where similar developments have occurred, some of them widely publicised in the media. As an education professional, it is important that you follow academic thinking on education issues as reported in textbooks and journals. This should enable you to think critically and decide how to interpret policy documents issued by the government and research findings released by renowned academic institutions on, for example, debates surrounding the teaching of English and maths in the primary classroom. These ideas link to sections 1.1 and 2.1 of the professional code of conduct issued by the Education and Training Foundation (nd; based on the Teachers' Standards, DfE, 2011):

- Develop your own judgement by reflecting on what works best in your teaching and learning to meet the diverse needs of learners (Teachers' Standard 5).
- Maintain and update your knowledge of educational research to develop evidence-based practice (Teachers' Standard 3).

In addition, you should also keep an eye on how these issues are reported in the media. As well as keeping you generally informed, it will also give you the opportunity to see issues from the parents' point of view – an idea of how they see education matters represented in the media.

Task

Exploring changes in thinking

1) How, to your knowledge, has general thinking developed on the following topics over time?

- Behaviour management
- Lesson planning and preparation
- Teaching SEND and EAL learners

- Pupil progress
- Safeguarding children in school
- Data protection

2) Can you identify any important academic studies in these areas?

3) How have these topics been reported on in the news media?

4) What, if anything, do you think needs to happen now in each case?

Advanced skills

Hegel's dialectic

A philosophical process called Hegel's dialectic quite nicely describes the advancement of knowledge in an academic environment. (Hegel was a nineteenth-century German philosopher; 'dialectic' is a formal word that essentially means 'discussion'.)

As illustrated in Figure 1.1, the dialectic basically states that for every **thesis** (ie idea) there will be an antithesis or antitheses (alternative idea[s]). Following a period of debate (which can last years, decades or centuries), a **synthesis** (a merging or fusing) of these ideas emerges. However, this new synthesis becomes a thesis in its own right and the process starts all over again!

Hegel's dialectic – how knowledge moves on

A two-way debate ensues that can last months, years or even centuries. The platform for debate is academic journals and conferences and, more recently, the internet

Scholars have ideas about the world and start testing and publicising these ideas

Other scholars start criticising and coming up with alternative ideas

THESIS debate ANTITHESIS

What often emerges from the debate is a synthesis where bits from both thesis and antithesis are accepted

SYNTHESIS

But the synthesis becomes a new thesis and so the process continues ... and knowledge moves forward!

Figure 1.1: Hegel's dialectic

Students at Level 4 (first-year undergraduate students) should be able to demonstrate understanding of one side of the debate. Most students grasp this relatively easily and soon realise that they will get good marks at this

CROSS REFERENCE

Appendix 1, Academic levels at university

academic level if they can convince the person reading (or marking) their work that they understand the concepts, ideas and theories they are writing about.

Level 5 (second-year) students are expected to be aware of the debate between ideas (thesis vs antithesis). Tied in with awareness of this debate is an understanding that there are alternative viewpoints, that there is always another side to the coin, and that if you are going to argue your corner, you must have evidence.

Being able to see how a compromise (synthesis) might be arrived at is a skill that Level 6 (third-year) students need to work towards and it is certainly a skill expected of postgraduate students. This skill is one that few beginners at university have – it's something most acquire as they climb the academic ladder.

At postgraduate level, synthesis is expected to a large extent in that most postgraduate work needs to be underpinned by original thought. This doesn't mean that you spontaneously make up your own theories; it usually means that you've appraised the viewpoints on a specific issue or topic and come up with your ideas about that issue or topic based on what you've read, digested and been convinced by.

Fake news!

The case studies previously discussed, on nappies and teaching of phonics, are important in that they show how knowledge and understanding change, and how academics, students and practitioners have a duty to avoid complacency and to keep asking questions. Unlike medicine, where new evidence emerges regularly with the potential of bringing about radical change, developments in education in the UK are not that explicitly marked by policy changes. The most influential reports which brought a radical shift in government policy may have been, perhaps, the 1967 Plowden Report (DES, 1967), published by the Department for Education and Skills (DES, 1967), and possibly the 1975 Bullock Report (DES, 1975). However, like health care, education is an important part of people's everyday lives, and so, notwithstanding the relatively slow pace of policy change, the public are likely be fairly attuned to ongoing debates in the media. It is therefore important for education students and professionals to appraise the media critically.

The concept of 'fake news' has come to the fore in recent years, and this has sometimes impacted on how educational policy has been viewed in some quarters. The concept of fake news comprises stories that have no basis in fact, but are nevertheless presented as factually accurate – often in order to benefit a particular person or organisation, but sometimes merely to cause mischief and controversy. They can appear in any medium but are particularly common on social media. Fake news stories often focus on politics and celebrity, but they sometimes involve education issues. The influence of this concept was recently highlighted when the *Collins Dictionary* named 'fake news' as the 2017 'word of the year' (Flood, 2017).

Task

Scrutinising the media

Look at the headlines below, taken from news media. Do you know the background behind these headlines? Do you think the stories could be classed as 'fake news'? Why? What questions need to be answered to get to the bottom of the story in each case?

Phonics method helps close attainment gap, study finds

(*The Guardian*, 25 April 2016)

Reading standards in England are best in a generation, new international test results show

(*The Telegraph*, 4 December 2017)

Is placing young children in ability groups 'a necessary evil'?

(*National Education Union Blog*, 18 December 2017)

Discussion of task

As with most headlines of this nature, there is actually a grain of truth in the ones cited above. Asking the right questions, however, means doing some detective work to determine if the underlying study or research may have been misinterpreted, or even distorted, by journalists or authors. You might even question whether the author or source has a particular political reason (most newspapers have a political stance) or financial reason (controversy breeds publicity!) for running the headline.

One way of probing headlines (or any other statement or claim) is to look for authoritative information on the subject. You might do this by checking out positions from legitimate scientific or professional organisations, or even consulting the original research that led to the headline. Indeed, as you progress through your education course, you will find more and more that this is what you are expected to do.

Phonics method helps close attainment gap, study finds

This headline from Weale (2016) puts two demands on a critically thinking education professional. Firstly, they should be aware of the dangers of possible misrepresentation or over-emphasis of the main argument and under-representation or trivialisation of any secondary or opposing arguments. An argument can be misrepresented if the focus is on certain findings while ignoring other equally relevant information. Here, the headline presents the argument that teaching reading using phonics results in long-term benefits for disadvantaged pupils from poorer backgrounds and those who do not have English as their first language. But, beyond the headline, which places sole focus on 'good news', the article also explains that, for other children, the use of phonics to teach reading brings no long-term benefits on average. The article reports that the benefits of phonics, while apparent at age seven, disappear at age eleven, suggesting that 'children who are not at a disadvantage will learn to read in any case'. So, while the headline focuses on the 'good news' about phonics, the article itself is much more circumspect. A critical reader needs to be aware of this potential disconnect between headlines and the articles accompanying them. The second demand on the critical professional is to track down evidence from reputable sources. In this case, as well as going directly to the research article cited, to make sure it has been accurately represented in the article, more up-to-date research on phonics, in relation to all children as well as economically disadvantaged and EAL children, should be investigated.

Reading standards in England are best in a generation, new international test results show

The article (Turner, 2017) relating to this headline refers to an international study (PIRLS) looking at the reading ability of nine and ten year olds in 50 countries. The study concludes that for the year 2017, England came in joint eighth place, which was the country's highest ranking since PIRLS was introduced in 2001. As with the phonics case study presented earlier in the chapter, through this article, it seems that the Conservative government of the time is taking credit for a policy (teaching of early reading through phonics) which was originally championed by the previous Labour government (1997–2010). Furthermore, this article makes use of emotive language such as 'winning the war' and 'pernicious arguments made by some academics', which has the effect of pitching the government, and even school teachers, against academics in higher education. Using these words or phrases unnecessarily can manipulate the reader's emotions. People tend to trust their own emotional responses and if an author can trigger an emotional response, then the reader is likely to be less critical of the reasoning. Hence, where subjects are emotive, it is particularly important to check the underlying reasoning carefully.

Is placing young children in ability groups 'a necessary evil'?

This is a headline published online as a blog on the National Education Union website in December 2017 (Heavey, 2017). The research underpinning this blog was conducted by Dr Alice Bradbury and Dr Guy Robert-Holmes from the Institute of Education (UCL) into ability groupings in Key Stage 1 and early years. The report found that the core subjects of literacy and maths and reading and phonics were the subjects where there was the most grouping. Phonics was seen as a discrete subject which is a special case, as the sequential nature of the government *Letters and Sounds* programme encourages grouping by 'phase' of phonics learning. As there is a dearth of recent research into the impact of ability grouping on the teaching of early reading through phonics, this report would seem welcome. However, it is important to remember that this report has been published as a blog. Although blogging is becoming a part of professional practice nowadays, it is very different from formal research reported in academic journals. Blog entries are generally informal, reflective, and moderate in length, and, importantly, they are not peer reviewed. Scientific findings and research can have far-reaching impact on society, in this case, on state education policies. It is therefore important that they undergo peer review, a process of quality control, before they are published and possibly impact on government policies. Furthermore, blogs can be impermanent, as individual posts or entire sites can be deleted without any notification to the reader, leaving no record of information cited. In this particular case, the same research has also been formally published (Roberts-Holmes and Bradbury, 2016) in a peer-reviewed journal with the title of 'The Datafication of Early Years Education and Its Impact Upon Pedagogy'. As a critical thinking teacher, you will be expected to consider the findings from the journal article, where, along with the findings, a rigorous argument based on a thorough literature review is presented, instead of relying on an online blog.

The need for critical thinking is apparent in all areas of public life. In the case study below, regarding a medical issue with many educational repercussions, critical thinking is related to 'scientific thinking' and contrasted to what is termed 'anecdotal thinking'.

Case study

Scientific versus anecdotal thinking

Shermer (2008) sees the public debate around vaccination and autism as symptomatic of the power of what he calls 'anecdotal thinking', and he suggests quite a compelling reason for this phenomenon:

The recent medical controversy over whether vaccinations cause autism reveals a habit of human cognition – thinking anecdotally comes naturally, whereas thinking scientifically does not. On the one side are scientists who have been unable to find any causal link between the symptoms of autism and the vaccine preservative thimerosal, which in the body breaks down into ethylmercury, the culprit du jour for autism's cause. On the other side are parents who noticed that shortly after having their children vaccinated autistic symptoms began to appear. These anecdotal associations are so powerful that they cause people to ignore contrary evidence: ethylmercury is expelled from the body quickly (unlike its chemical cousin methylmercury) and therefore cannot accumulate in the brain long enough to cause damage. And in any case, autism continues to be diagnosed in children born after thimerosal was removed from most vaccines in 1999; today trace amounts exist in only a few. The reason for this cognitive disconnect is that we have evolved brains that pay attention to anecdotes because false positives (believing there is a connection between A and B when there is not) are usually harmless, whereas false negatives (believing there is no connection between A and B when there is) may take you out of the gene pool.

(Shermer, 2008)

Developing and applying your critical thinking skills

Critical thinking is not peculiar to academia or education practice: people are required to use their critical faculties every day in order to make assessments, judgements and decisions. However, in academic and education settings, your critical thinking skills will be under particular scrutiny. You will need to consciously develop your critical thinking skills throughout your study and practice, and you will need to draw on these skills in order to complete academic tasks successfully and develop as a teacher. This will involve a range of skills and abilities which you will have to draw on at different stages of your studies and work:

- problem solving, including discussion of ethical issues;
- decision making;
- applying objective criteria to particular situations;

CROSS
REFERENCE

Chapter 3,
Critical
reading

- reflecting on your education practice and on your study skills;
- analysing and evaluating sources of information and ideas in terms of suitability, quality and relevance;
- analysing and evaluating information in order to understand a topic;
- identifying, interpreting and assessing the position of other people;
- identifying, interpreting and assessing the arguments put forward by other people to determine if
    - they are well thought through
    - they are reasoned and balanced
    - they are supported with sound, relevant evidence
    - they lead to logical conclusions;
- identifying, interpreting and assessing contrasting points of view;
- evaluating the strength and relevance of the evidence put forward to support different points of view;

CROSS
REFERENCE

Chapter 4,
Critical
writing

- using academic sources to develop your own position (or 'stance') in relation to the topics you will investigate, and presenting (or 'voicing') this stance in a way that will convince a critical reader;
- developing arguments to support your stance which are well thought through, reasoned and balanced;
- finding sound, relevant evidence to support your arguments.

All of the above are explored in later chapters in this book.

Critical thinking in education practice

Critical thinking is inherent in the Teachers' Standards (Part 1 and 2) issued by the Department for Education (DfE, 2011) in England, which outline how a teacher is expected to demonstrate consistently high standards of personal and professional conduct. The Education and Training Foundation outlines the following professional skills (based on the Teachers' Standards) which reflect the importance of critical thinking in key areas of teaching practice.

Teachers and trainers are reflective and enquiring practitioners who think critically about their own educational assumptions, values and practice in the context of a changing contemporary and educational world. They draw on relevant research as part of evidence-based practice.

1. Professional attributes and values:

   1.1 Develop your own judgement by reflecting on what works best in your teaching and learning to meet the diverse needs of learners (Teachers' Standard 5).

   1.2 Avoid assumptions and promote social and cultural diversity, equality of opportunity and inclusion (Teachers' Standard 5).

   1.3 Evaluate and challenge your practice, values and beliefs.

2. Professional knowledge and understanding:

   2.1 Maintain and update your knowledge of educational research to develop evidence-based practice (Teachers' Standard 3).

   2.2 Evaluate your practice with others and assess its impact on learning by working with mentors and peers (Teachers' Standard 8).

   2.3 Demonstrate an objective ability to apply theoretical understanding of effective practice in teaching, learning and assessment drawing on research and other evidence.

3. Professional skills:

   3.1 Apply appropriate and fair methods of assessment and provide constructive and timely feedback to support progression and achievement (Teachers' Standard 6).

   3.2 Enable learners to share responsibility for their own learning and assessment, by giving regular feedback and setting goals that stretch and challenge (Teachers' Standard 6).

   (Education and Training Foundation, nd)

Task

Applying the Teachers' Standards to critical thinking

1) Research has shown that children of poorer parents display substantially worse maths and reading skills than their peers by the time they start primary school. Other studies have revealed that these wide gaps in pre-school skills persist into adulthood and help explain low educational attainment and lifetime earnings. So, it is often claimed that there isn't much that teachers can do in school to raise achievement for all children. How would you respond to such a mentality? Should teachers have high expectations? Why?

2) The benefits of 'mindfulness for children' in primary schools have been much discussed in the media in recent years. Would you recommend this practice to the parents and children in your school?

Discussion of task

The numbers in brackets are cross-references to the sections of the Professional Teachers' Standards (DfE, 2011) mentioned earlier.

1) Think about the Teachers' Standards when considering the issue.

- Be careful not to make assumptions when discussing terms like 'aspirations' and 'expectations', which have subtle, but very important, distinctions (1.2). Aspirations are about wanting to be better, whereas expectations convey a belief about the likelihood of success. Raising expectations has been proven to help pupils, but the same can't be said for aspirations.

- Analyse the research evidence, for example, on aspirations, which found that 'interventions which aim to raise aspirations have little to no positive impact on educational attainment' (Aspirations Interventions EEF, 2018) (2.1). A recent study (Khattab, 2015) found that students who have high aspirations, but low expectations, are twice as likely to get fewer than five GCSEs at A*–C than their peers who have both high aspirations and high expectations.

- Explore ways of helping children and parents by making explicit your expectations for the children at the start of the school year or at the beginning of new tasks and topics. Get parents involved, as parents play a huge role in shaping how young people see themselves. Encourage high self-expectations in students who do not see themselves in a positive light, as it can be very helpful to create a culture of growth mindset (Inner Drive, nd) (3.2). Make sure that your suggestions are evidence based (2.1), that they take account of individual needs and abilities of children, and that you monitor the situation to track the effects of your intervention.

2) Mindfulness can mean many things, from a formal, evidence-based intervention like Mindfulness-Based Stress Reduction or Mindfulness-Based Cognitive Behaviour Therapy to informal commercial courses or groups based on Buddhist practices. However, it is worth noting that much of the recent growth of interest in well-being and mindfulness in schools in the UK is coming less from an education perspective and more from public health officials concerned about growing mental instability among young people (1.1, 1.2). An example recommendation, compatible with the Teachers' Standards, would be something like:

There is research evidence indicating that the age of onset of clinical depression is getting lower and lower. Mindfulness, yoga and meditation have all been growing in popularity in schools around the country as a way to support pupils' wellbeing and mental health. However, there are multiple factors feeding into mental health issues, for example, poverty. Willem Kuyken, a professor of clinical psychology at Oxford University and director of the Oxford Mindfulness Centre, has urged caution about the widespread adoption of the practice in schools (Kuyken et al, 2015). Bearing this in mind, it is advisable to analyse the evidence base (2.1) before you recommend it to your school or parents. For example, check the findings of the Mindfulness in Schools Project (nd), led by Oxford University, and *Mindful Nation UK*: Report by the Mindfulness All-Party Parliamentary Group (MAPPG, 2015).

Reflection

1) Try to think of more incidences where the aspects of the Teachers' Standards discussed in the previous section would be applicable.

2) Think of any practical steps you could take to ensure you follow the guidelines.

3) What **questions** might you want to ask (and to whom) to help you take the best course of action?

Applying critical thinking to ethical issues

As a teacher, you will encounter many difficult situations and it is important that you respond in a way which is both informed and objective. You will be expected to approach these situations critically, to question when necessary, to analyse and evaluate each situation, and to provide reasoned argument to support the position you adopt. It is also necessary to listen to arguments of others involved in the situation, and to appraise them critically.

Task

Critically appraising ethical concerns

Look at case study A below, based on a real-world referral, and answer the questions which follow.

Case study A

A Year 2 girl was repeatedly upset and began to seek comfort in her male class teacher. She would come to him for a hug each time something happened that made her cry or feel sad. Over time, she showed signs of being more settled at school, but although these episodes were getting fewer, she still sought comfort about once every week or so. The teacher tried to suggest that, since she was doing so well, maybe the next time she was upset, she didn't come for a hug but was a big girl and dealt with it herself. She went home and complained that Mr Smith used to give her lots of hugs, but said that he wouldn't any more, and the very angry and concerned mother contacted the school.

Do you think the teacher's actions were based on critical thinking?

What responses/actions/proactive measures based on critical thinking might result in a more positive outcome?

Discussion of case study A

According to the guidelines issued by the National Education Union (2013) about physical contact with pupils:

> It is not illegal to touch a pupil. There are occasions when physical contact, other than reasonable force, with a pupil is proper and necessary.

> Examples of where touching a pupil might be proper or necessary include:

- when comforting a distressed pupil
- when a pupil is being congratulated or praised
- to demonstrate exercises or techniques during PE lessons or sports coaching
- to give first aid.

However, touch can be interpreted differently based on social customs and personal perspective. What is acceptable and pleasant to one person may be unacceptable and even distressing to another. Male teachers are advised not to touch or pat a child even to comfort them, but, instead, to ask a female colleague to step in, if necessary. Also, when having to reprimand a child, they should do so with the classroom door open or in the earshot/view of another member of staff, ideally female. In this case, this male teacher should have informed the senior management about the issue right from the start and dealt with it by following guidance from the management. So, in this instance, the male teacher did in fact lack critical insight when acting to comfort an upset pupil.

Task

Critically appraising ethical concerns

Look at case study B below, and answer the question that follows.

Case study B

> In a Year 9 science lesson, one child, Bill, is being particularly disruptive and running around the room, interfering with the practical work of other groups. He constantly shouts at others and is creating havoc in what is an otherwise productive lesson. The teacher asks him to leave the room and cool off for a moment, but the pupil refuses. The teacher stands by the door and asks Bill to come over and speak to him. As he comes over, the teacher places a hand in the small of Bill's back and guides him through the now open door. As he does so, Bill shouts out 'Get off me! I'm telling my dad you assaulted me! That's child abuse!', and runs off down the corridor. The teacher returns to the classroom and continues with the lesson.
>
> Do you think the teacher's actions were based on critical thinking?

Discussion of case study B

According to the guidelines issued by the National Education Union (2013), teachers in both England and Wales have a statutory power to use reasonable force to restrain pupils in a number of circumstances, as set out in Section 93 of the Education and Inspections Act 2006. The DfE guidance on the Use of Reasonable Force provides that teachers can use reasonable force:

- to remove disruptive children from the classroom where they have refused to follow an instruction to do so
- to prevent a pupil behaving in a way that disrupts a school event or a school trip or visit
- to prevent a pupil leaving the classroom where allowing the pupil to leave would risk their safety or lead to behaviour that disrupts the behaviour of others
- to prevent a pupil from attacking a member of staff or another pupil, or to stop a fight in the playground
- to restrain a pupil at risk of harming themselves through physical outbursts.

When removing a child physically from the classroom, teachers should do so in the presence of a member of the senior leadership team. Furthermore, schools should train all teachers in 'Team Teach physical handling training', which can be found at www.teamteach.co.uk. Only teachers who have been trained to handle such situations should be put into such a position.

In this case, the teacher did lack some critical insight when he placed a hand in the small of Bill's back and guided him through the open door.

Reflection

Our views of what education should look like and how it should materialise depend on our own experience of it and our personal values. While some campaigners argue that education should be firmly rooted in the personal and intellectual development of young people, there are others who believe that more emphasis should be placed on making schools and teachers more accountable through national curriculum requirements and corresponding statutory assessments, creating an education system more fit for the economy in the twenty-first century. Teachers have a responsibility to view the government's education policies critically. They also have a responsibility to use their knowledge and critical skills to identify questionable practice in schools and act accordingly.

1) What are your own views on the role of education? How do you think you came to hold these opinions?

2) What action could you take if you spotted something which concerned you in your placement area or workplace?

Top tips

Exploiting opportunities to hone your critical thinking skills

1) Seminars are an important part of teaching and learning in universities. They are a way of checking your knowledge and understanding, and usually relate directly to lectures and assessments. Importantly, they can provide a space for you to develop your critical thinking skills. They can provide a great opportunity to question others and to test your own ideas in preparation for essays and presentations.

2) Exercise your mind by playing 'devil's advocate'. If your instincts seem to lead you to a particular point of view, try to find arguments and evidence to support the other side. You may not change your mind, but your position will be stronger because you will have tested it.

3) Always try to find the assumptions that lie behind any position. Ask yourself if these assumptions need to be questioned.

4) Don't equate authority or confidence with reason: an authoritative or confident person may be right or wrong. Judge them on the *facts*.

Summary

This chapter has explored the nature of critical thinking in academia and education with reference to real-life case studies. It has focused on the importance of questioning and reasoned argument, and it has introduced strategies for developing and applying critical thinking skills. It has highlighted the centrality of critical thinking in the Teachers' Standards and in education practice. The following chapters further explore these issues.

References

Aspirations Interventions, EEF (2018) *Teaching and Learning Toolkit* [online]. Available at: https://educationendowmentfoundation.org.uk/evidence-summaries/teaching-learning-toolkit/aspiration-interventions/#effectiveness (accessed 18 February 2019).

Collins, S (2015) The Nappy Science Gang That Took on the NHS. *The Guardian*, 30 November [online]. Available at: www.theguardian.com/science/sifting-the-evidence/2015/nov/30/nappy-science-gang-versus-the-nhs (accessed 5 March 2018).

Department for Education (2011) *Teachers' Standards* [online]. Available at: www.gov.uk/government/publications/teachers-standards (accessed 7 March 2019).

Department for Education and Skills (1967) *Children and their Primary Schools* (The Plowden Report: Report of the Central Advisory Council for Education in England) London: HMSO.

Department for Education and Skills (1975) *A Language for Life* (The Bullock Report) London: HMSO.

Education and Training Foundation (nd) *Professional Standards for Teachers and Trainers – England* [online]. Available at: www.et-foundation.co.uk/supporting/support-practitioners/professional-standards (accessed 7 March 2019).

Flood, A (2017) Fake News Is 'Very Real' Word of the Year for 2017. *The Guardian*, 2 November [online]. Available at: www.theguardian.com/books/2017/nov/02/fake-news-is-very-real-word-of-the-year-for-2017 (accessed 5 March 2018).

Heavey, A (2017) Is Placing Young Children in Ability Groups 'a Necessary Evil'? *National Education Union ATL Section* [Blog] [online]. Available at: www.atl.org.uk/latest/placing-young-children-ability-groups-%E2%80%9C-necessary-evil%E2%80%9D (accessed 17 January 2019).

InnerDrive (nd) How Do You Actually Develop a Growth Mindset [Blog] [online]. Available at: https://blog.innerdrive.co.uk/how-do-you-actually-develop-growth-mindset (accessed 3 March 2019).

Khattab, N (2015) Students' Aspirations, Expectations and School Achievement: What Really Matters? *British Educational Research Journal*, 41(5), 731–48.

Kuyken,W, Hayes, R, Barrett, B, Byng, R, Dalgleish, T, Kessler, D, Lewis, G et al (2015) Effectiveness and Cost-Effectiveness of Mindfulness-Based Cognitive Therapy Compared with Maintenance Antidepressant Treatment in the Prevention of Depressive Relapse or Recurrence (PREVENT): A Randomised Controlled Trial. *The Lancet*, 386(9988), 63–73.

MAPPG (2015) *Mindful Nation UK: Report by the Mindfulness All-Party Parliamentary Group*. London: The Mindfulness Initiative.

Mindfulness in Schools Project (nd) [online]. Available at: https://mindfulnessinschools.org (accessed 3 March 2019).

National Education Union (2013) *Lecture Notes: Education, the Law and You* [online]. Available at: www.teachers.org.uk/members-reps/new-teachers/education-law-and-you (accessed 7 March 2019).

Roberts-Holmes, G and Bradbury, A (2016) The Datafication of Early Years Education and Its Impact upon Pedagogy. *Improving Schools*, 19(2), 119–28 [online]. https://doi.org/10.1177%2F1365480216651519

Shermer, M (2008) Wheatgrass Juice and Folk Medicine [online]. Available at: https://michaelshermer.com/2008/08/wheatgrass (accessed 5 March 2018).

Simpson, D (2017) More Mindful Schools? [online]. Available at: www.danielsimpson.info/archive/mindfulness-in-schools-constructive-critique (accessed 25 January 2019).

Turner, C (2017) Reading Standards in England are Best in a Generation, New International Test Results Show. *The Telegraph* [online]. Available at: www.telegraph.co.uk/education/2017/12/04/phonics-revolution-reading-standards-england-best-generation (accessed 17 January 2019).

Warburton, N (2012) *A Little History of Philosophy*. New Haven, CT; London: Yale University Press.

Waugh, D (2014) Phonics Test Results are a Credit to the Last Government. *The Guardian* [online]. Available at: www.theguardian.com/education/2014/sep/25/phonics-test-results-credit-government (accessed 10 January 2019).

Weale, S (2016) Phonics Method Helps Close Attainment Gap, Study Finds. *The Guardian* [online]. Available at: www.theguardian.com/education/2016/apr/25/phonics-method-helps-close-attainment-gap-study-finds (accessed 17 January 2019).

Chapter 2
Reflective practice

Learning outcomes

After reading this chapter you will:

- understand what is meant by the terms 'reflection' and 'reflective practice';

- understand how reflection and reflective practice are an inherent part of critical thinking;

- have gained insight into a number of models of reflective practice and be able to apply them critically;

- be familiar with the characteristics of reflective writing and be able to produce reflective writing which demonstrates these characteristics.

CROSS
REFERENCE

*Studying for
your Education
Degree,*
Chapter 3,
Becoming
a member
of your
academic and
professional
community,
The education
community,
Reflective
practice

CROSS
REFERENCE

*Studying for
your Education
Degree,*
Chapter 6,
Assessment

Reflection is the critical analysis of a situation or event, focusing on your own experience, perceptions, behaviour and thought processes. It is a way of making sense of your experience and relating it to your wider studies and professional development.

Practice-based disciplines like teaching have long promoted reflection and regarded it as an important aspect of critical thinking. What's more, reflection is gaining increasing importance across all academic subjects. You will notice that in this book there are a number of 'reflection' tasks which require you to think about your own experiences, abilities and beliefs. These tasks have been included because we, the authors, believe that reflection forms an important part of studying, and of critical thinking in particular. Your assessments at university may include reflective essays and shorter accounts/weekly reflections which may form part of your professional portfolio or reflective journal. This chapter will help you to develop your reflective skills and thus enhance both your education studies and your teaching practice.

Reflection and reflective practice

In education, you will be expected to reflect on your experience of practice, positive and negative, and to write about it. Teachers are expected to develop into reflective practitioners and reflection is also an essential part of Initial Teacher Training (ITT) as outlined in the Teachers' Standards. Teachers' Standard 4 states that teachers must 'reflect systematically on the effectiveness of lessons and approaches to teaching'(DfE, 2011, p 11). Reflective practice is a tool used to enhance the performance of practitioners, through, for example, reflecting on and rectifying previous mistakes.

Through reflection, you will be expected to demonstrate a developing understanding of your practice so that you grow as a practitioner. This may involve better understanding of:

- how to select or adapt/change resources;
- differentiation levels;
- behaviour management;
- inclusion for SEND/EAL children;
- how to meet the needs of all children in the class;
- how to work better with colleagues and schools;
- decision making and solving problems.

Reflection

1) What experience do you have so far of reflective activities in your studies or of reflective practice? How did you feel about these experiences?

2) Do you think of yourself as a naturally reflective person, or do you find reflection difficult?

Reflective frameworks

There are a number of reflective models designed to help students think things through in a structured manner. In education, there are three which are widely used:

- Brookfield's four lenses model (2017);
- Gibbs' reflective cycle (1988);
- Johns' model of structured reflection (1995).

Brookfield's four lenses model

Brookfield emphasises reflecting through four lenses:

1) Self – personal experiences

2) The students' eyes

3) Colleagues' perceptions

4) Academic research

He appreciates the use of all four lenses to create an inclusive action plan. This model utilises the reflector's feelings, their pupils' view point, what their peers have said/will say and what literature/theories support the reflection. Brookfield's model helps us apprehend how reflective practice in teaching is inclusive in nature as it examines how the teacher's performance affects not only themselves but their pupils and peers. The combination of self-reflection, student feedback and peer assessment can, for example, enable a recognition of hidden habits one may not recognise alone (Brookfield, 2017).

To be critically reflective, practitioners need to step outside of themselves, and Brookfield's four different viewpoints provide a framework within which to do this. Indeed, understanding the students' perspective is paramount in teaching and relationship building (and key in managing behaviour for learning); and exploring actions through the lenses of colleagues and academic theory contributes to teachers' professional development, as outlined in the DfE Teaching Standards (DfE, 2011). More importantly, Brookfield demands a thorough examination of assumptions and of the way practitioners interact with each other within the community of practice. In order to be critically reflective, teachers need to ask whose interests are served by particular codes of practice and stay alert to the way in which they are embracing ideas and behaviours that may or may not be subtly harming them.

Gibbs' reflective cycle

Gibbs' reflective cycle is a well-known and widely used reflective framework. It was heavily influenced by **Kolb's learning cycle** (Kolb et al, 1991), a way of explaining how people learn through experience. This concept is known as **experiential learning**.

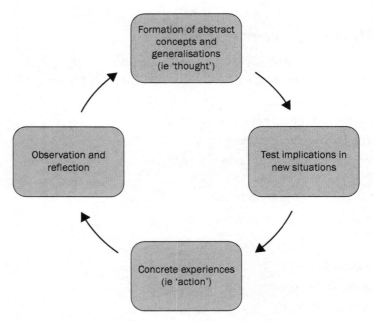

Figure 2.1: Kolb's learning cycle (adapted from Kolb et al, 1991, p 59)

Kolb argues that learning is a **cyclical process** involving a continuous dialogue between thoughts and actions (or theory and practice), mediated by two processes: testing and reflection. In other words, in experiential learning, you test out your ideas in practice, reflect on what goes well and not so well, readjust your ideas if need be, and subsequently test them out. Importantly for practice-based disciplines like teaching, Kolb's model implies that students will struggle to link theory to practice effectively without reflective skills.

Kolb's learning cycle has been highly influential in higher education, and many teachers and students find it very useful. However, like any theory, it must be viewed critically, and, in fact, some scholars have criticised it for being somewhat simplistic, selective and lacking in empirical support. See Tennant (1997) for views on both sides.

Gibbs' model (influenced by Kolb) is also cyclical.

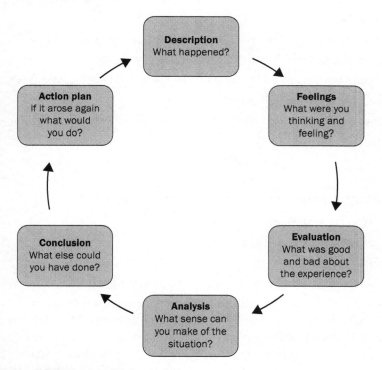

**Figure 2.2: Gibbs' reflective cycle
(adapted from Gibbs, 1988, p 50)**

Gibbs' model has six stages, all of which (except perhaps description) require a degree of critical thought or analysis about the particular situation you are interested in. For example, the 'feelings' stage requires you to note how you feel (angry, upset, overjoyed, anxious, etc) and then think about whether the feelings were appropriate, or perhaps an under- or over-reaction; the 'analysis' stage is about you trying to make sense of the situation; and the 'conclusion' stage is about exploring whether there were alternative ways to deal with the situation.

Johns' model of structured reflection

Johns' model of structured reflection is based on five cue questions which enable practitioners to break down their experience and reflect on the process and outcomes. Johns (1995) used Barbara Carper's (1978) patterns of knowing in nursing as the basis for his model, exploring aesthetics, personal knowing, ethics and knowledge accumulated through observation and experiment. He added reflexivity (connecting with previous experiences) as a way of understanding how an experience can change and improve practice.

This model focuses on the following five cues:

1) Description of the experience

What happened and what were the significant factors which affected the situation?

2) Reflection

What was I trying to achieve and what are the consequences?

3) Influencing factors

What things like internal/external knowledge affected my decision making?

4) Could I have dealt with it better?

What other choices did I have and what were the consequences of my actions?

5) Learning

What will change because of this experience and how I felt about the experience?

How has this experience changed my ways of knowing?

- Empirics – scientific
- Ethics – moral knowledge
- Personal – self awareness
- Aesthetics – the art of what we do, our own experiences

Johns' model (2000) offers a very detailed framework for reflection and shares some similarity with Gibbs' model (1988) with regard to examining our emotion at the time of the event. As well as the description of the event and examination of our emotions, there is analysis of the factors surrounding the event, and possible alternative responses/actions. In addition, there are further thoughts on how you arrived at that decision-making process – through reflexivity, or what Johns calls 'empirics'. Through this process, education professionals can start to unpick, examine and understand core elements of their practice that may have previously gone unchallenged.

Critically evaluating reflective frameworks

The reflective models outlined in the previous section have different approaches, but cover a lot of the same ground. It is useful to analyse the models and compare their approaches and terminology in order to establish which, if any, will work best for you.

Task

Comparing and contrasting reflective frameworks

Look back at the descriptions of the three reflective models outlined in the previous section and, using Brookfield's four lenses model as a starting point, complete a table like the one below with comparable elements where possible.

BROOKFIELD'S FOUR LENSES	GIBBS' REFLECTIVE CYCLE	JOHNS' MODEL
eg personal experiences	What happened? What did you think/ feel?	experience, reflection

Now that you have analysed the three models, you are better placed to evaluate them so that you can decide how useful they will be to you in your study and practice.

Task

Evaluating reflective frameworks

List the strengths and weaknesses of each model and relate them to your own learning style or preference. In the third column, you may wish to consider which model might work better for you in a given situation: Brookfield's model, which encourages reflection from multiple perspectives, Gibbs' cyclical model or Johns' linear one.

	STRENGTHS	WEAKNESSES	RELATION TO PERSONAL PREFERENCES
Brookfield			
Gibbs			
Johns			

CROSS
REFERENCE

Studying for your Education Degree, Chapter 2, Strategies for effective learning, Learning styles

Reflection-*in*-action and reflection-*on*-action

Reflection-on-action involves professionals reviewing and analysing past incidents to gain new understanding, with the aim of improving future practice. Reflection-in-action requires that professionals explore incidents, and their reaction to incidents, as they occur.

In education circles, Schön's work on reflective practice, Educating the Reflective Practitioner (1983) is regarded as a seminal text. In it, he distinguishes between reflection on action and reflection in action. Reflection on action is something that occurs after an event; reflection in action is something that occurs during the event. The former is a necessary skill for any practitioner; the latter is a deeper skill which can enable fuller development. Finlay (2008) attributes Schön's promotion of 'professional artistry' over technical rationality through reflection-in-action as an attempt to develop truly reflective practitioners. This goes deeper than merely applying a model for the process of reflection. Schön (1983) argues that real-life practice is complicated and unpredictable, and that professionals need to do more than just follow a check-list or a set procedure – they need to draw on their practical experience as well as theory, and thus engage in a creative process. Schön (1983) compares it to the improvisation of a jazz band and also notes that reflection is a dialogue between thinking and doing through which the participant becomes more skilful.

Reflection on learning

It is important that you identify and benefit from the many opportunities at university to reflect on your own learning, and that you use these to improve your knowledge, understanding and performance.

CROSS REFERENCE

Studying for your Education Degree, Chapter 6, Assessment, Feedback on academic work

One frequently overlooked opportunity is **feedback** from lecturers or even peers. This could include oral feedback in class or a tutorial, or written feedback on a piece of writing. Writing feedback from a lecturer could be on a first writing draft to help you make improvements before you hand it in, or it could be to explain and justify the mark you were given for an assessment. It is important that you are open to feedback, which will be easier if you manage not to take criticism too personally; it is also important that you take time to analyse and reflect on feedback, and that you use it to develop. Feedback from peers can also be helpful, especially if you are working collaboratively on a group presentation or report; just be careful that collaboration doesn't turn into something which could be interpreted as collusion.

School supervision

Reflection is an essential part of Initial Teacher Training (ITT) in that it comprises part of the Teachers' Standards. These are legislative documents which set out the minimum level of practice expected of teachers and trainee teachers, and Teachers' Standard 4 states that teachers must 'reflect systematically on the effectiveness of lessons and approaches to teaching' (DfE, 2011, p 11) as part of their practice.

The guidelines issued by the current government state that all accredited ITT providers must ensure that training programmes are designed to provide trainee teachers with sufficient time being trained in schools, early years and/or further education settings to enable them to demonstrate that they have met all the standards for QTS. Hence, training programmes are structured to include time in educational settings ranging between 24–32 weeks depending upon the duration of the actual programme.

Education training courses set out to help education professionals develop and reflect on teaching skills, so that they can learn from their experiences. Learning from experience, described by Schön (1983) as 'reflective practice', is an important teaching trait. Student teachers are learners, and like the pupils they teach, they need knowledgeable others to help them on this journey. In order to observe quality teaching, student teachers need to be placed in an environment that encourages learning and where the experienced teachers serve as exemplars of good practice and provide clear supervision and mentoring.

The importance of supervision for student teachers should not be underestimated. Supervision should involve processes that promote the involvement of student teachers in reflection and action, which are believed to have the most successful outcomes (Gibbs, 1996). Often, school-based mentors support education practitioners during their time in school. These mentors can be: school-based tutors jointly appointed by the university to supervise students on school-based practice and experience; proactive senior colleagues engaged in actively training new teachers without an evaluative role (Heath-Camp and Camp, 1990); resource persons, problem solvers, evaluators and providers (Godley, 1987); exemplars – successful teachers who work on upper grade levels and subject matter and who work in close proximity to the new teachers.

Reflection will take many different forms, including: lesson evaluations; weekly journals or diary entries; post-lesson observation discussion with tutors, class teachers, mentors and examiners; academic essays; discussions during taught sessions in the university.

Writing reflectively

As an education professional, you will be expected to write reflectively in a number of assessments. You may be required to write reflective essays or provide short weekly reflective accounts, often for your professional portfolio. Some modules may require you to complete a reflective diary, sometimes called a journal or log. Student teachers are often asked to use the reflective models described earlier in this chapter to help them reflect on their experiences and organise their ideas in writing.

Short written reflections

In this section, you will analyse short written reflections which would typically appear in an education student's professional portfolio or reflective journal.

CROSS REFERENCE

Academic Writing and Referencing for your Education Degree, Chapter 1, Academic writing: text, process and criticality, Writing short reflections for journals and portfolios

Task

Identifying appropriate and effective reflections

Read the following written reflections. Which ones are more appropriate and effective? Why?

1) This week, as part of the starter activity, I gave the students an assignment-type worksheet to test whether they had learnt the material from last week. Upon marking, I realised that there were some students that were still stuck on the material that I had taught them the previous week. It's hard work! I'll have to start all over again.

2) Last week during one of my first maths lessons, I overran considerably as the lesson went on for longer than planned. This was partly because the class took every opportunity to talk, which resulted in me then having to regain control. My inexperience also led me to play it very safe in my lesson. I took a very behaviourist approach, not allowing for any real pupil involvement and instead making them copy out what was written on the board for most of the lesson.

3) The importance of being able to see the behaviour of students from the students' viewpoint was highlighted while I was observing a Year 10 citizenship class. During this class, it became apparent that a couple of students in the class were of a facetious disposition, often trying to jest with the teacher. But when I started to teach the class myself, instead of condemning this type of behaviour, I decided to embrace the jokey comments, which I think enabled the lesson to go back on track. The class teacher agreed with me.

4) In one school incident, a student – who had been taken out for intervention – refused point blank to engage in any learning during our one-to-one class. Being a one-to-one session, I was able to be flexible in my approach to teaching and adopt a number of different strategies, but still to no avail. It was only through gentle discussion and questioning that I was able to prise from the student that he disliked being singled out for intervention, taken out of art (his favourite lesson), and having no control over which lesson he missed.

5) Once I combined the two reflective models, Gibbs (1988) and Brookfield (1995), I recognised my personal feelings had got in the way in this situation, which had led me to make assumptions. My aim had been for the lesson to be enjoyable and engaging for all students, including B. However, when I later came to reflect on the range of activities I had given the class as a whole. I realised they were quite analytical and heavy. My action plan, informed by Gardner's 'changing practice' (2010), resulted in creating a subsequent lesson which was engaging yet effective, one which every student would enjoy. Once this plan was put into action, B was one of the most engaged students in the next lesson – which surprised both the class teacher and me.

6) The EAL lead gave a helpful CPD session after school, which she recommended for me to attend. Before the next lesson, I analysed my situation, explored ways to adapt the learning for M, and produced an action plan to enhance this child's learning.

7) During an observation of PSHE for Year 8, the teacher I was observing got really irritated by the behaviour of two particular pupils, and after some time, he called one an 'idiot' and he sent the other one out. Do I want to become a teacher that says that to her students? I know I don't, but will it ever slip out of my mouth?

8) Today, while teaching a PSHE lesson about drugs awareness, I encountered a few personalities. Let's be real, it is impossible to have a perfect class, so it is important to be aware of the challenges we might face. Last week, during my mentor meeting, I got what I consider one of the best pieces of feedback for behaviour management and behaviour for learning: joke with them – if they make a joke about the topic, or say something when they shouldn't, or say something that they know is wrong (but not disrespectful), follow their lead. You will not make a change or gain their trust by ignoring the fact or simply saying: that's wrong or inappropriate. Sometimes it is good to use their comments as part of the lesson and use them to your advantage.

Discussion of task

1) This reflection focuses on lesson planning. Here, the student's reflection is overly reliant on description and lacking in evaluation regarding the focus of reflection. Furthermore, there should be connections made between personal assumptions, habits or values and the focus of reflection. It should end by indicating how the reflection will direct future actions.

2) This reflection is focused on pupil engagement in lessons and the challenges that come along. There is an appropriate depth of thought given to how the experience made the student feel, and the student has demonstrated how their learning might be enhanced by the experience.

3) This reflection is focused on behaviour management. Here, the student teacher took a risk that worked well based on his/her understanding of the situation. Now, the teacher should develop their understanding of various behaviour theories and approaches so that their actions are based on in-depth understanding of behaviour management.

4) In this instance, Brookfield's model is extremely useful in reflecting as the student teacher needed to view the situation from the perspective of the student. No amount of outstanding lesson planning or pedagogy could have coaxed this student into co-operating. Brookfield's model provides a useful and powerful tool for daily reflection as it offers the opportunity to reflect from different perspectives. The consideration of multiple points of view allows us to deepen our reflection.

5) This reflection focuses on lesson planning and resourcing. It is successful because feelings are analysed, viewpoints are acknowledged, and the student tries to connect it all to their learning and development.

6) Here the student clearly thinks about the situation, listens to other people's points of view, and tries to pull these together to work out how learning might be enhanced as a consequence.

7) Verbal abuse by teachers can be an overwhelmingly negative experience for children. Here the teacher seemed to have developed a dysfunctional strategy to deal with the pressures of the classroom. However, the root cause may lie in teacher stress and burn-out. In order to combat teacher stress and burn-out, training should be made available to help teachers adapt to their role and develop the personal capabilities necessary to meet the demands of their profession. From the student's perspective, gathering more information about various needs and abilities will help the student to understand the pressures of the profession and develop resilience as a result.

8) This is a good reflection because the focus is on matching the 'reality' to the expectations of being a teacher. It also shows that the student is receptive to noticing the things that students value.

Top tips

Preparing to write reflections

CROSS REFERENCE

Academic Writing and Referencing for your Eduation Degree, Chapter 1, Academic writing: text, process and criticality, Writing essays, Reflective essays

1) Consider the **purpose** of the reflection.

2) Use a **reflective model** or framework (such as Brookfield's, Gibbs' or Johns') if it helps you organise and deepen your reflection. Adapt the model to suit your own learning preferences.

3) Keep **clear records**, maintaining **anonymity** throughout.

4) Decide the right **time** to write up your reflection – leave enough time for you to have some distance between you and the situation or event, but not so much time that your memory is negatively impacted.

Longer written reflections and essays

In this section, you will analyse a longer written reflection which might typically form part of a reflective essay.

Task

Analysing reflective writing

Read the reflective account below and analyse it with reference to the reflective models described earlier in the chapter.

There are many models for reflection, and through critically exploring the value of reflective practice, I concluded that Brookfield's (2017) model, combined with Johns' (1995) questioning cues, offered the most analytical framework for self-examination. Adopting Kolb's (1984) active experimentation completes my chosen framework, bringing together critical self-reflection that can crystallise into positive change.

Without behaviour for learning, there can be no learning – a powerful lesson

Behaviour management proved a key struggle in my first placement, and I spent a large proportion of my time reflecting on this, identifying and examining factors that led to poor classroom behaviours; I considered how my lack of experience, and inconsistency in implementing school policy, fuelled this outcome. Guided by Brookfield (2017) to consider theoretical approaches to behaviour management, I came to appreciate the value of behaviourism, which I had previously viewed as too blunt an instrument for modern learning. In re-examining the value of behaviourism, and re-questioning my assumptions, I realised that the reward and sanction system put forward by Skinner's (1974) operant conditioning theory formed the basis of many schools' behaviour policy, and in turn, would formulate mine.

Initially, I was reluctant to reprimand forcefully or issue detentions, and reflected deeply to understand why this was. I was uncomfortable with my own perception of 'strict teachers', which was based on personal experience of students being shouted at, and ultimately humiliated, and the teacher losing control – all undesirable outcomes. However, extensive observation of other teachers enforcing school policy revealed that this perspective was far from the current reality. This highlights the weakness of the single viewpoint in Kolb's (1984) model.

Under Brookfield (2017), I was able to reframe my idea of a strict teacher from a negative construct to a positive one that consistently enforced the school's behaviour policy to the benefit of students' learning, and to dismantle my internal construct, which equated negative emotions with losing control. Moreover, I came to fully appreciate the importance of classroom management and behaviour-for-learning, because in their absence, learning is impossible.

Fairness ranks highly in my values, and in reflecting on those values, I saw the injustice in how my poor behaviour management negatively impacted on other staff. Through active experimentation with different strategies informed by theories and colleagues – using tone, direct speech and body language, giving praise, tactically ignoring attention-seeking behaviours, engaging with pupils, as well as issuing detentions when necessary (Ellis and Tod, 2015; Rogers, 2015) – I became more consistent and able in my behaviour management. This impacted positively on students' learning.

I found the results of this particular reflection both powerful and empowering because it altered my perceptions about myself and allowed me to express my emotions in a constructive way, thereby enabling students to 'read me'. The process also tapped into my personal ambition of changing lives through education.

Reflection on how children learn

To make the most of my classroom observations, I sought to systematically unearth learning theories that underpinned those lessons, research into those theories, and reflect on their adaptation in observed classes, before considering which elements to incorporate into my own practice.

During these observations, I saw constructivist approaches being adopted. This concept rejects the idea, posed by behaviourism, of knowledge being passively received. Under the constructivist paradigm, teachers create a learning environment that enables students to construct their own understanding of the world, shifting the focus from teacher to student, with my function more as a facilitator, prompting, asking probing questions and providing the necessary scaffold to guide students' learning. Bruner (1960), Piaget (1977) and Vygotsky (1978) are among the key protagonists of this school of thought in focusing on assimilation and accommodation of new ideas into an existing framework. Applefield et al (2001) outlines constructivist principles, explain how they can be implemented and counter some of the myths around them.

Guided by this theory, I promoted discovery learning, problem-solving and group work in my lessons, encouraging students to actively think about their learning, compare and contrast ideas, and incorporate ideas in a way that makes sense to them. Students have different ways of 'seeing' a problem, and the act of sharing and discussing not only facilitates learning, but also encourages students to take ownership of it (Applefield et al, 2001). However, this approach requires/assumes that there is a solid knowledge base in which new learning can be assimilated, and/or that students are suitably motivated (Brophy, 1999; Sivan, 1986).

Through reflection-in-action and reflection-on-action, I learnt that introducing a completely new topic in mathematics using constructivism led to misconceptions becoming embedded as most students relied on methods which were self-taught. As a result, many pupils were confused or overwhelmed by the work, lacking the sufficient cognitive skills to formulate their new learning or problem-solve. I, of course, take responsibility for not sufficiently scaffolding the work, but at times, the scaffolding requirements were so great and diverse that I was forced to revert to direct teaching. Indeed, problems remained even after ensuring I had understood pupils' pre-existing knowledge – as outlined by the DfE Teaching Standards 2 – to appropriately scaffold activity.

More importantly, Kirschner et al (2006) found that most controlled studies favoured direct, strong instructional guidance over constructivist-based methods. Armed with this knowledge, I concluded that constructivist approaches were most effective after students had built up a suitable repertoire of domain-specific knowledge/schemas (Tricot and Sweller, 2014). As a result, I altered my strategy, and found the combination of direct teaching, modelling and chunking learning created less confusion and better student outcomes/behaviours. Additionally, by building in active and deep questioning and discussions that allow for formative assessments (Black and Wiliam, 1998), students were not merely passive recipients of knowledge. Only when a core understanding is developed would I consider implementing purely constructivist techniques.

<u>Conclusion</u>

The deep thought processes involved in reflection leave me in no doubt of its importance in my development – as a way of thinking and being, thus ensuring that I will continue to grow and remain dynamic in my practice.

Through critical reflection, I am now more able to: look for and be open to different perspectives and meanings; examine uncomfortable truths; and formulate solutions that are informed and evidence-based to the benefit of students.

Discussion of task

The reflection corresponds to many elements of the reflective models (Brookfield, 2017; Gibbs, 1988, Johns, 2009) discussed earlier in the chapter. There is:

- **Description** of a particular situation in the first half of the reflection (placement in a school) and the feelings that arose in the student ('I was uncomfortable with my own perception of "strict teachers"', 'I found the results of this particular reflection both powerful and empowering'). There is then a description of a critical incident (behaviour management) and the student's immediate reaction to and feelings about the incident (re-examining the value of behaviourism, re-questioning assumptions). In the second half, the student teacher also explored honestly how her personal theories of learning had a considerable influence on her interpretation in the first half of the reflection constructivist theories of learning (scaffolding the maths activity).

- Insightful **analysis** and **evaluation** of the outcomes of the incident itself identified problematic issues underlying theoretical models. For example, there were learning opportunities provided by the experiences of the teachers implementing school behaviour policy and from challenges posed when implementing constructivist theories in the scaffolding of the maths task. It is clear from this writing that the student has been open and honest about her journey as a reflective practitioner. Research into reflection and the aspects of teaching and learning that the student has focused on demonstrate excellent research skills. In addition, she has been able to synthesise complex material and it is evident that her own 'self' as a teacher is emerging. The writing moves between description of the teaching process, analysis of the student's feelings and developing understanding through engagement with research.

- Effective **analysis** of the **follow-up** to the incident and the **learning experiences** gained by seeking feedback from more experienced teachers. For example, through engagement with theories underpinning behaviour management and feedback from mentors, the student found the results of this particular reflection both powerful and empowering because it altered her perceptions about herself.

- **Implications for future practice**: greater consistency in behaviour management and judicious implementation of constructivist approaches; ability to look for and be open to different perspectives and meanings, openness to examination of uncomfortable truths, and ability to formulate solutions in future teaching practice.

The language of reflection

Writing reflectively requires command of a particular style of writing, which is in some ways different from the style of writing you will be asked to use in other critical essays.

Reflection

What do you notice about the type of language used in the reflections you have studied in the previous section?

Discussion of reflective language analysis

Reflective writing is characterised by a number of features:

CROSS REFERENCE

Appendix 2, Verb forms in English

- A range of tenses, eg the past tense (simple, continuous, perfect) to describe the incident or experience ('I spent a large proportion of my time reflecting on this'; 'I was reluctant to reprimand forcefully'; 'I altered my strategy'); the present tense (simple, continuous, perfect) to describe current feelings and beliefs ('Fairness ranks highly in my values'; 'teachers create a learning environment'); the future tense to describe planned action ('ensuring that I will continue to grow'; 'would I consider implementing constructivist techniques').

- A slightly conversational tone ('I had previously viewed as too blunt an instrument for modern learning'; 'I sought to systematically unearth learning theories').

- The first-person pronoun ('make the most of my classroom observations'; 'I was forced to revert to direct teaching').

Task

Identifying useful words and phrases

Match the headings (1–5) to the sets (A–E) of phrases below, taken from the previous reflective essay.

1) Reflection on current knowledge and attitudes;

2) Describing feelings;

3) Highlighting important points;

4) Signalling how the situation or event has challenged previous thinking;

5) Impact on practice.

A

More importantly, …

Indeed, …

B

… I had previously viewed as too blunt an instrument …

… revealed that this perspective was far from the current reality.

… it altered my perceptions …

… I learnt that …

C

… proved a key struggle in my first placement …

Initially, I was reluctant to …

I was uncomfortable with …

D

… I came to fully appreciate …

… I was able to reframe my idea of …

… I became more consistent and able in ….

This impacted positively on students …

I am now more able to …

E

... ranks highly in my values ...

... in reflecting on those values ...

Top tips

Language bank

Make a note of language which will help you to signal and organise the different aspects of your reflection, perhaps adding phrases to a diagram of the reflective model you are using (see Figure 2.3 as an example). Start with the phrases in Figure 2.3 and Table 2.1 below, which add to and expand on the language discussed in the previous task.

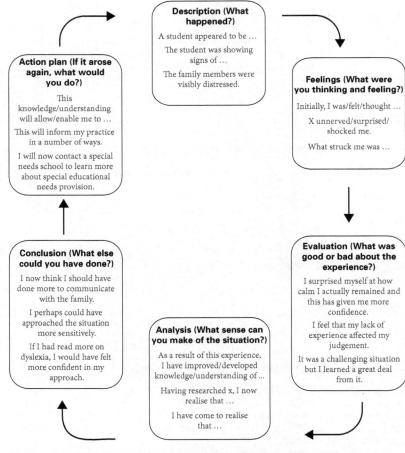

Description (What happened?)

A student appeared to be ...

The student was showing signs of ...

The family members were visibly distressed.

Action plan (If it arose again, what would you do?)

This knowledge/understanding will allow/enable me to ...

This will inform my practice in a number of ways.

I will now contact a special needs school to learn more about special educational needs provision.

Feelings (What were you thinking and feeling?)

Initially, I was/felt/thought ...

X unnerved/surprised/shocked me.

What struck me was ...

Conclusion (What else could you have done?)

I now think I should have done more to communicate with the family.

I perhaps could have approached the situation more sensitively.

If I had read more on dyslexia, I would have felt more confident in my approach.

Evaluation (What was good or bad about the experience?)

I surprised myself at how calm I actually remained and this has given me more confidence.

I feel that my lack of experience affected my judgement.

It was a challenging situation but I learned a great deal from it.

Analysis (What sense can you make of the situation?)

As a result of this experience, I have improved/developed knowledge/understanding of ...

Having researched x, I now realise that ...

I have come to realise that ...

Figure 2.3: An example of a reflective model with language cues added

Table 2.1: The language of reflection

Reflection on current/previous knowledge and attitudes		
I	don't know/understand much/enough about … tend to …	

| Prior to this,
 Previously, | I | had thought that …
 hadn't been aware of … |

Describing feelings		
(Initially,)	I	was … felt/was feeling … thought …

Describing reactions to a situation or incident	
X	unnerved me surprised me shocked me made me panic made me nervous/uncomfortable/guilty struck me as …

My immediate reaction was to …

One of the things that What Something that	struck me immediately was … surprised me was … shocked me was …

Highlighting important points			
For me, the most	important significant useful	occurrence event issue	was …

Significantly, …   Importantly, …   Crucially, …   In fact, …   Clearly, …

Signalling how the situation or event has challenged previous thinking				
As a result of this experience, Subsequently,	I have	improved developed improved enhanced	my	knowledge of … understanding of … skills in … ability to …

Having	analysed discussed read researched	x,	I now	feel … know … understand …
I have	realised that … come to realise that … begun to understand …			

Impact on practice			
This	knowledge understanding	will	allow me to … enable me to … inform my practice

Top tips

Beating writer's block!

Sometimes, you may find yourself staring at a blank page, not quite knowing how to start. Don't worry too much about this – you are not alone; it happens to everyone from time to time. The important thing is to have strategies to overcome this writer's block. One thing that can help is to actually start with some key phrases, such as those given in the previous sections, and use these to prompt your own ideas. **The meaningful nature of many of these phrases will also help you to shape your ideas in a more critical way.**

Summary

This chapter has explored the concepts of 'reflection' and 'reflective practice' and their place in critical thinking. It has presented key models of reflective practice and provided opportunities to analyse and evaluate them so that you can determine if and how they will support your own reflective practice. It has highlighted the key distinction between reflection *in* and reflection *on* practice. It has discussed the importance of reflecting on your learning and emphasised the key role of feedback. The chapter has also introduced the important concept of 'school supervision'. Finally, it has provided some linguistic tools to help you write reflectively.

References

Applefield, J M, Huber, R and Moallem, M (2001) Constructivism in Theory and Practice: Toward a Better Understanding. *High School Journal*, 84(2), 35–53.

Black, P and Wiliam, D (1998) *Inside the Black Box: Raising Standards through Classroom Assessment.* London: School of Education, King's College, University of London.

Brookfield, S (1995) *Becoming a Critically Reflective Teacher*. San Francisco: Jossey-Bass.

Brookfield, S (2017) *Becoming a Critically Reflective Teacher*. 2nd ed. San Francisco: Jossey-Bass.

Brophy, J (1999) Toward a Model of the Value Aspects of Motivation in Education: Developing Appreciation for Particular Learning Domains and Activities. *Educational Psychologist*, 34(2), 75–85.

Bruner, J S (1960) *The Process of Education*. Cambridge, MA; London: Harvard University Press.

Carper, B (1978) Fundamental Patterns of Knowing in Nursing. *Advances in Nursing Science*, 1(1), 13–23.

Department for Education (DfE) (2011) *Teachers' Standards* [online]. Available at: www.gov.uk/government/uploads/system/uploads/attachment_data/file/665520/Teachers__Standards.pdf (accessed 1 February 2019).

Ellis, S and Tod, J (2015) *Promoting Behaviour for Learning in the Classroom: Effective Strategies, Personal Style and Professionalism*. London; New York: Routledge.

Finlay, L (2008) Reflecting on Reflective Practice. *PBPL CETL, Open University* [online]. Available at: www.open.ac.uk/opencetl/resources/pbpl-resources/finlay-l-2008-reflecting-reflective-practice-pbpl-paper-52 (accessed 1 February 2019).

Finlayson, A (2015) Reflective Practice: Has It Really Changed over Time? *Reflective Practice*, 16(6), 717–730. doi:10.1080/14623943.2015.1095723

Gibbs, G (1988) *Learning by Doing: A Guide to Teaching and Learning Methods*. Oxford: Further Education Unit, Oxford Polytechnic.

Gibbs, C (1996, October) Enhancing Student Teaching through Interventionist Supervisory Strategies. Paper presented at the *New Zealand Council for Teacher Education Conference*, Palmerston North, New Zealand.

Godley, L B (1987) The Teacher Consultant Role: Impact on the Profession. *Action in Teacher Education*, 16(1).

Heath-Camp, B and Camp, W (1990) What New Teachers Need to Succeed. *Vocational Education Journal*, 65(4).

Johns, C (1995) Framing Learning through Reflection within Carper's Fundamental Ways of Knowing in Nursing. *Journal of Advanced Nursing*, 22, 226–34.

Johns, C (2009) *Becoming a Reflective Practitioner*. 3rd ed. Chichester: Wiley.

Kirschner, P A, Sweller, J and Clark, R E (2006) Why Minimal Guidance During Instruction Does Not Work: An Analysis of the Failure of Constructivist, Discovery, Problem-Based, Experiential, and Inquiry-Based Teaching. *Educational Psychologist*, 41(2), 75–86.

Kolb, D (1984) *Experiential Learning: Experience as the Source of Learning and Development*. Upper Saddle River, NJ: Prentice Hall.

Kolb, D, Rubin, I and Osland, J (1991) *Organisational behaviour: an experiential approach*. 5th ed. London: Prentice-Hall International.

Northern Illinois University, Faculty Development and Instructional Design Center (2010) Howard Gardner's Theory of Multiple Intelligences [online]. Available at: www.niu.edu/facdev/_pdf/guide/learning/howard_gardner_theory_multiple_intelligences.pdf (accessed 16 May 2019).

Piaget, J (1977) *The Essential Piaget*. London: Routledge and Kegan Paul.

Rogers, B (2015) *Classroom Behaviour: A Practical Guide to Effective Teaching, Behaviour Management and Colleague Support*. 4th ed. Los Angeles: SAGE.

Schön, D (1983) *The Reflective Practitioner: How Professionals Think in Action*. New York: Basic Books.

Sivan, E (1986) Motivation in Social Constructivist Theory. *Educational Psychologist*, 21(3), 209–33.

Skinner, B F (1974) *About Behaviourism*. London: Jonathan Cape.

Tennant, M (1997) *Psychology and adult learning*. 2nd ed. London: Routledge.

Tricot, A and Sweller, J (2014) Domain-Specific Knowledge and Why Teaching Generic Skills Does Not Work. *Educational Psychology Review*, 26(2), 265–83.

Vygotsky, L S (1978) *Mind in Society: The Development of Higher Psychological Processes*. Cambridge, MA: Harvard University Press.

Chapter 3
Critical reading

Learning outcomes

After reading this chapter you will:

- be better able to select academic sources for assignments which are both credible and relevant;

- understand more about how to engage critically with sources;

- know more about how to analyse and evaluate arguments and evidence in sources effectively.

In order to complete assignments at university, you will be required to access the literature relevant to your discipline, mostly in the form of textbooks and academic journals. This chapter guides you towards understanding which sources are suitable for the task in hand. It discusses how to engage critically with the literature, how to go about analysing and evaluating the arguments and evidence presented so that you can develop and support your own position in oral and written assignments.

Selecting sources for an assignment

A university assignment, whether it is an academic essay or presentation, is, in many ways, an account of your own critical journey through the literature as you form your position with regard to a particular topic or issue. In academia, this position is often known as your 'stance'.

Your stance is expressed through your argument, and a good argument must draw on and engage with sources that both have credibility in an academic context and are directly relevant to the assignment task or question in hand.

Top tips

Identifying possible sources

Textbooks can be a useful starting point. They can provide an overview of a discipline (eg mathematics in primary schools) or a topic (eg managing pupil behaviour), outlining and illustrating current ideas, beliefs and evidence. They may also summarise the way in which knowledge and understanding in that area has evolved over time, pinpointing any changes in direction regarding the main issues or debates.

CROSS REFERENCE

Studying for your Education Degree, Chapter 5, Academic resources: technology and the library, The university library

▲ **Journal articles** often advance a particular position and argument. This is usually based on a piece of primary research carried out by the authors, but it could also be built around a systematic review of major studies conducted by others. Note that journal articles, which have been subject to a review by an expert panel of referees, are considered to be more academic than articles in periodicals, which tend to be chosen by the editor. Note also that there is a hierarchy of journals and periodicals, with some carrying more weight than others. Influential journals have what is known as a high **impact factor** (Garfield, 2006), and, the more you progress in your studies, the more you will be expected to draw on these weightier journals. Your university library will help you to identify and access appropriate journals by providing access to databases which are important in education, such as ERIC (Education Resources Information Center), Web of Science and PsycINFO. You can usually access these databases through electronic interfaces such as OVID, EBSCO and ProQuest.

Top tips

Reading efficiently

There are limits on the time you can devote to reading, so it is very important to read efficiently. In order to decide if an article will be relevant, you might want to work your way down the list below, putting the article aside as soon as it seems that it may not be relevant to the task, thereby saving precious reading time:

1) the title;
2) the abstract or summary;
3) the keywords (if included);
4) the introduction;
5) the conclusion;
6) the whole article.

Note that a well-written title and abstract may give you all the information you need in the first instance.

Selecting credible sources

In order to assess the *credibility* and *authority* of a source, you should pose a set of critical questions:

- Who wrote/created it? Is the author an academic authority in the field? If an organisation, what type of organisation is it? (A respected professional body, the government, a charity, a corporation?)
- Is it published by a reputable academic publisher/journal?
- What is the author's purpose in writing? (To inform, argue a particular position, sell products?)

- Who is the intended reader or listener? (Students, other scholars, potential customers?)
- Is this source cited by other credible scholars?
- Is it a recent publication? Is this fact relevant/important – do later publications draw on new evidence, or advance the argument in any way, for example?
- What is the scope of the work? Is it comprehensive, or is it limited in some way?

Selecting relevant sources

It is important to be able to establish that a source has credibility in an academic sense; however, to be of any use to you in an assignment, a source must also be *relevant*. It is not enough that a source is merely connected to the topic in hand; relevance can only be established with precise reference to your precise **purpose** in writing or presenting, and this entails careful analysis of the assignment task or question. This initial 'unpacking' of the task requires careful, *critical* reading.

Task

Unpacking the task

Look at the following Level 5 essay-writing tasks and identify the following (discussed later in the chapter):

- the general **topic**;
- the particular **focus** of the assignment;
- any **instruction words** which tell you how to **approach** the assignment.

A

Outline current practice in assessing children's acquisition of phonics skills and critically evaluate the extent to which these are effective for all children.

B

Critically evaluate public and political perceptions of the role of the teacher and perceptions of the impact teachers can have upon pupils' learning.

Task

Assessing the relevance of journal articles

Look at the following extracts (title, abstracts, keywords, plus some extracts from introductions) from journal articles and decide if and in what way they might relate to the essays in the previous task.

CROSS REFERENCE

Academic Writing and Referencing for your Education Degree, Chapter 1, Academic writing: text, process and criticality, The writing process, Approaching a writing assignment

CROSS REFERENCE

Academic Writing and Referencing for your Education Degree, Chapter 1, Academic writing: text, process and criticality, The writing process, Analysing a writing assignment

CROSS REFERENCE

Appendix 1, Academic levels at university

1)

Title
Assessing reading development through systematic synthetic phonics

Abstract
This narrative literature review evaluates the effectiveness of synthetic phonics in comparison with analytic phonics. It presents the key research findings and offers a critical appraisal of this research. Primary schools have developed a variety of assessment processes which assess pupils' knowledge and skills in synthetic phonics. It is through using these assessment tools that gaps in pupils' knowledge and skills are identified and these gaps then form the basis of subsequent synthetic phonics interventions. The article concludes by arguing that a more detailed assessment framework may be required for the purpose of assessing children's reading development than the model which schools currently adopt.

Introduction
This narrative literature review evaluates the effectiveness of synthetic phonics in comparison with analytic phonics. It presents the key research findings and offers a critical appraisal of this research. For over a decade now, and following the publication of the Rose Review in 2006 (Rose, 2006), educational policy in England has emphasised the need for schools to provide children with a systematic programme of synthetic phonics instruction. In synthetic phonics children learn to read by identifying the smallest units of sound within a word (phonemes) and blending these together to read the target word. It is different from other approaches to phonics which focus on blending larger units of sound.

The emphasis on synthetic phonics has been embedded in the Teachers' Standards (DfE, 2011) in order to ensure that all teachers have good knowledge of synthetic phonics. The Teachers' Standards were developed by the Department for Education (DfE) in 2011 to provide a framework for identifying the minimum standards expected of all teachers. In addition, inspection frameworks for both initial teacher education providers and schools have been revised several times since 2006 and these revisions have resulted in inspectors paying increasing attention to the teaching of synthetic phonics in schools.

Schools have developed a variety of assessment processes which assess pupils' knowledge and skills in synthetic phonics. It is through using these assessment tools that gaps in pupils' knowledge and skills are identified and these gaps then form the basis of subsequent synthetic phonics interventions. For some children synthetic phonics is highly effective in enabling them to master the skill of decoding. This provides them with a strategy for reading unknown words. However, for others the approach is less effective. For example, dyslexics sometimes struggle to master the skill of decoding and instead rely on whole word recognition strategies. This raises a question about whether an alternative approach to learning to read would be more beneficial for pupils who have difficulty processing sound at the level of the phoneme. For these children alternative methods of assessing their reading development and teaching them may be necessary.

Although logic suggests that one size does not fit all, the emphasis on synthetic phonics in the Teachers' Standards suggests quite the opposite. Thus, even if early assessments indicate that the approach is not successful, the political endorsement of synthetic phonics in the Teachers' Standards suggests that teachers should persevere with this approach by providing systematic synthetic phonics intervention programmes for those children who are falling behind. This is deeply worrying, given that subsequent further failure can impact detrimentally on children's self-concept.

This article examines two approaches to phonics to identify which is the more effective. It concludes by arguing that a more detailed assessment framework may be required for assessing children's reading development.

(Glazzard, 2017)

2)

Title
Decoding the phonics screening check

Abstract
The statutory 'phonics screening check' was introduced in 2012 and reflects the current emphasis in England on teaching early reading through systematic synthetic phonics. The check is intended to assess children's phonic abilities and their knowledge of 85 grapheme–phoneme correspondences (GPCs) through decoding 20 real words and 20 pseudo words. Since the national rollout, little attention has been devoted to the content of the checks. The current paper, therefore, reviews the first three years of the check between 2012 and 2014 to examine how the 85 specified GPCs have been assessed and whether children are only using decoding skills to read the words. The analysis found that out of the 85 GPCs considered testable by the check, just 15 GPCs accounted for 67% of all GPC occurrences, with 27 of the 85 specified GPCs (31.8%) not appearing at all. Where a grapheme represented more than one phoneme, the most frequently occurring pronunciation was assessed in 72.2%

of cases, with vocabulary knowledge being required to determine the correct pronunciation within real words where multiple pronunciations were possible. The GPCs assessed, therefore, do not reflect the full range of GPCs that it is expected will be taught within a systematic synthetic phonics approach. Furthermore, children's ability to decode real words is dependent on their vocabulary knowledge, not just their phonic skills. These results question the purpose and validity of the phonics screening check and the role of synthetic phonics for teaching early reading.

Keywords
phonics; grapheme–phoneme correspondences; reading; decoding.

(Darnell et al, 2017)

3)

Title
Researching 'teachers in the news': the portrayal of teachers in the British national and regional press

Abstract
An outline of frameworks for conceptualising and analysing news media roles in the representation of teachers is followed by a discussion of quantitative and qualitative approaches to the study of news coverage. An argument is made for the benefit of using corpus linguistic tools within the overall conceptual focus on lexical and syntactical structures offered by critical discourse analysis. Findings are presented from a comprehensive study of the press portrayal of teachers and education. Focusing on the portrayal of teachers in news headline coverage, the study shows a considerable lexical and syntactic change between 1991 and 2005 in the public/news representation of teachers, broadly from a negative view of teachers as troublesome to a more positive emphasis on teachers as a hardworking profession besieged by mounting pressures.

Keywords
news coverage; teacher images; longitudinal news analysis; framing; corpus linguistics; critical discourse analysis

Introduction
The media, both national and local, are an important public arena for the articulation and contestation of education issues and professional identities. Concern about the media's role in shaping and influencing public images of teachers and education is neither particularly recent

(e.g. Ball 1990; Wallace 1993), nor is it a particularly British phenomenon (e.g. Blackmore 2004; Maeroff 1998). But while numerous studies have examined the portrayal of teachers in film and other entertainment media content (e.g. Dalton 2003; Ellismore 2005), including the mapping of changes in such images over time, there have been surprisingly few longitudinal studies of that most prominent and politically important genre of media content: news.

Important exceptions to this dearth of longitudinal research are Matilda Wiklund's research on how representations of teachers in a leading Swedish newspaper have changed since the early 1980s (Wiklund 2003), and Peter Cunningham's (1992) study of changing British press presentations of teachers and education over the years 1950, 1970 and 1990. Such mapping of changing media images provides an important component for examining the relationship between changes in media images and changes in public perceptions, as established for example through regularly conducted opinion surveys.

(Hansen, 2009)

4)

Editorial
The importance of teachers, teaching and school leaders: the 'silver thread' of the reform agenda for English schools

It has become evident that primary schools in England are struggling to appoint headteachers with over a quarter of schools with a vacancy forced to re-advertise and with a particularly severe problem in London where nearly half of all headteacher posts have to be readvertised (TES 2013a). The work of this writer can attest to the fact that this is not a new phenomenon since large-scale studies of the challenges in developing senior leaders carried out in the late 2000s revealed that there was a 'potential leadership crisis' (Rhodes, Brundrett, and Nevill 2008) and that government agencies needed to assist schools in asking key questions such as: What creative mechanisms can we use to encourage staff to aspire to leadership roles?; and, How do we know we really are a good training ground for leadership talent development? (Rhodes and Brundrett 2008, 23). If this potential crisis intensifies one must conjecture what this may mean with a national agenda for education that puts ever greater stress on the role of the headteacher in enhancing school effectiveness.

(Brundrett, 2013)

CROSS
REFERENCE

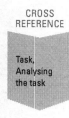

Task,
Analysing
the task

Discussion of tasks

You first need to think carefully about the words you highlighted earlier in the chapter, related to topic, focus, and instruction:

A

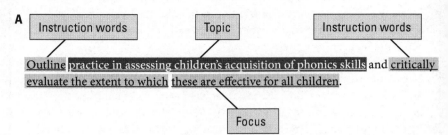

The extracts from Paper 1 indicate that this article is highly relevant to the topic. The study is based upon a review of relevant literature rather than an empirical study by the author. This kind of meta-analysis, whereby academics look at a range of studies, can be very helpful in offering readers a broad perspective on a topic. The article was published in 2017 and so is quite up to date and able to focus on current assessment, particularly via the phonics screening tests over a few years since their inception. The paper explores assessment of children with different needs, such as those with dyslexia, and is therefore relevant to the focus of the essay.

Paper 2 provides considerable detail on the nature of the phonics screening test and questions whether its content is appropriate for testing different skills involved in reading. The paper also looks at the nature of the grapheme-phoneme correspondences (GPCs) which are tested and so provides technical knowledge about phonics and children's acquisition of phonic skills. The paper was published in 2017 and so may be felt to be up to date. However, it reviews the first three years of the phonics screening check between 2012 and 2014 and readers will need to ascertain whether there have been changes to the test since then when critically evaluating its effectiveness for all children.

B

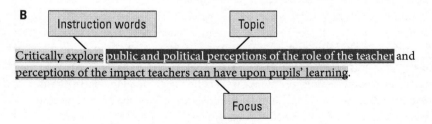

Paper 3 is potentially very useful for this assignment as it draws upon research which is highly relevant to the topic. However, it was published in 2009 and draws upon research which focuses on the period 1991 to 2005, so it is possible that later studies may have found that perceptions of teachers may have changed. Further study of other texts will be needed to enable an informed discussion of perceptions of teachers' impact on pupils, as that is not the focus of Hansen's paper.

Paper 4 is an editorial from an academic journal. It is potentially useful for this assignment as it provides an overview of what were then current developments. While it is quite recent, it should be borne in mind that school education is constantly changing in response to government legislation, so it would be important to seek more recent sources too. However, the paper does focus on a significant period of change, and on the Secretary of State's comments about teachers and the teaching profession, so it is relevant. It is important to bear in mind that editorials express the editor's opinions and, while these may be informed by the content of other articles in the journal, they are not necessarily developed through first-hand research.

Engaging critically with sources

The work that you produce on your degree programme should be informed and enhanced by the literature. You should therefore read with an eye to doing more than merely reproducing the ideas and arguments of others in word-for-word notes. Such a 'knowledge-telling' approach (Beirerter and Scardamalia, 1987) could ultimately lead to your own work ending up as a mere 'patchwork' of ideas, and you will probably be criticised for being overly descriptive and uncritical. It is therefore necessary to *engage critically* with the literature, and to adopt a 'knowledge-transforming' approach (Beirerter and Scardamalia, 1987); this means scrutinising and synthesising the ideas, arguments and evidence you encounter as you read, with a view to using them to develop your own position.

CROSS REFERENCE

Chapter 4, Critical writing, What does it mean to write critically?

Scrutinising

As you note and relate the arguments and evidence you encounter, it is important to scrutinise them, asking questions as you read:

- Is an argument based on sound reasoning?
- Is there sufficient evidence to support the argument?
- Is the evidence credible and convincing?
- Has evidence (or alternative interpretations of evidence) which might counter the argument been given due consideration?

Synthesising

Reading critically means being careful not to look at facts, ideas, arguments, evidence, findings, conclusions etc in isolation. The critical reader is alert to any trends, patterns or relationships which emerge as they read across the literature, and is conscious of anything which may not fit these. The ideal is to find ways to represent these things in your notes as you encounter them, organising the ideas and evidence you discover, so that you are already preparing to say something about how *you* understand and interpret the current state of knowledge. (In Chapter 4 of *Studying for your Education Degree*, there is an example of how note-taking (in this case on the relative merits of different approaches to teaching reading) can develop in a focused, critical fashion.)

CROSS REFERENCE

Studying for your Education Degree, Chapter 4, Critical thinking, Applying and developing your critical thinking skills, Synthesis of information and ideas

It is also vital to constantly relate what you find in the literature with your particular context, ie the task or question you are working on.

CROSS
REFERENCE

Chapter 4,
Critical writing,
What does it
mean to write
critically?

Telling your research story

As noted earlier, the academic work you produce is in some ways the story of your journey through the literature, an account of how your own thought processes have developed as you encountered, analysed and evaluated the ideas and arguments of scholars in the field. This is the essence of **originality** (and the antithesis of *plagiarism*!), as the journey you have been on is unique to you, and only you can tell this story. This individual and unique **voice** is what makes your essay different from other people's essays. If you approach the reading and writing process with this in mind, your voice should grow to be mature and confident.

Task

Being a critical reader

Read the extracts below (taken from the journal articles introduced earlier in the chapter) and answer the questions. (The questions are aimed at helping you to read critically.)

A

An effective assessment battery in reading should include an assessment of the pre-reading skills identified above. It should include the development of auditory and visual discrimination, phonological awareness and visual memory. It is only through developing a more detailed assessment battery which assesses children's pre-reading skills that teachers will then be able to target the teaching to match the area of need for those children whose word reading skills are not secure by the age of 7. Within each of these areas there are subcomponent skills which need to be assessed. It is possible that intervention through a phonics-only approach will compound a sense of failure and result in teaching which is not developmentally appropriate. Different types of teaching and more comprehensive assessment batteries need to be developed to address different stages of development in reading. Given the inconclusive evidence in relation to synthetic phonics, an assessment tool which only assesses children's skills in this aspect of phonics, such as the phonics screening check, is not fit for purpose.

(Glazzard, 2017, pp 52–3)

Questions

1) What key concepts are introduced in this extract?

2) What do you understand them to mean?

3) In what way are they relevant to essay A (discussed earlier in the chapter)?

B

Summary and conclusions

News coverage of teachers and education features prominently in both national and regional newspapers. Newspapers are thus an important public arena for definitions of what the key issues, challenges and tasks facing education and teachers are, as well as potentially a key source of public definitions of the identity and status of teachers. While it would be foolhardy to think of the role of news-definitions of teachers and education in terms of 'direct impact' on political, public or teachers' own perceptions of the status of teachers, the analysis presented here shows the reservoir of public images from which such perceptions may draw. The study's retrospective analysis of the portrayal of teachers from 1991 to 2005 shows a considerable and important change from a largely negative to a largely positive portrayal of teachers.

There was much explicitly positive or supportive reporting of teachers, increasingly so towards the latter end of the 1990s and through 2005, and not infrequently casting teachers as 'heroically' fighting against extraordinary outside pressures on them, the education system and on students. The identifier 'teacher' itself was shown to carry powerful positive connotations. While much coverage focused on confrontation between teacher unions and government or government related institutions, there was markedly less emphasis on confrontation – and concomitantly more emphasis on support and help to teachers – in the most recent period.

The misconduct of individual 'bad' teachers was highly newsworthy and consequently figured prominently in the headlines, but it was extremely rare to find headlines which showed teachers – as a body of professionals – as anything other than dedicated and committed professionals struggling against a broad range of serious problems and pressures. Earlier news coverage of the teacher bashing mould (Ball 1990, Wallace 1993, Woods et al 1997) has given way to a more supportive and less confrontational style of reporting, which gives teachers a prominent voice and recognises, as genuine, the problems and pressures faced by teachers.

Methodologically, the analysis sought to combine the recognised analytical strengths of critical discourse analysis (particularly its twin focus on lexical choice and syntactical structures) with the computer-assisted tools and strengths of corpus linguistics. The latter concerned particularly the ability to reliably identify the occurrence and context of selected key-words in large and representative bodies of text, as well as the ability to systematically make transparent for analysis important changes over time. The tracking of changes in words associated with the keyword 'teacher(s)' (collocation analysis) and the ability (with the help of concordance software) to view all occurrences of the keywords in their immediate context combined to systematically reveal important lexical and syntactical shifts, over the period analysed here, in the way teachers are referred to and characterised in newspaper discourse. The mapping of such shifts in news coverage in turn provides a context for understanding important changes in public and political – as well as teachers' own – perception of the status and condition of teachers.

In summary, the study showed that the image of teachers and the teaching profession changed and improved considerably between the early 1990s and 2005. While there was, due to the intrinsic news-value of such stories, a great deal of headline coverage of 'bad' individual teachers in sexual and other misconduct cases, teachers – as a professional body – were increasingly portrayed in a way which implied respectability and esteem, which afforded recognition to their claims, and which recognised their plight and (sometimes) beleaguered situation as a genuine problem requiring political action.

(Hansen, 2009)

Questions

1) What does the author mean by 'public definitions of the identity and status of teachers'?

2) What sort of 'evidence' of changes in news coverage of teachers is presented here?

3) What research methodology did the author use to analyse changing perceptions of teachers in the media?

4) What might be problematic about using this kind of data?

Discussion of task

A

1) Concept clarification is an essential part of good essay-writing. In this paper, a key concept is that different types of teaching and more comprehensive assessment batteries need to be developed to address different stages of development in reading.

2) The author identifies auditory and visual discrimination, phonological awareness and visual memory as key elements in reading. These can be explained within an essay.

3) Essay A asks that current practice in assessment be critically evaluated and that a critical evaluation of their effectiveness for all children be made. The paper clearly addresses both of these elements.

B

1) The 'public definitions of the identity and status of teachers' are those reflected in what was seen in newspaper headlines and articles.

2) and 3) The author used computer technology to analyse lexical choice (words used) and syntactic structures (grammar/phrasing) associated with the word 'teacher[s]' over a period of time and then analysed these in order to draw conclusions about changing perceptions.

4) Although newspaper articles were analysed electronically, the interpretation of the results relies upon personal interpretation by the author, which might be affected by preconceived ideas about teachers and teaching. The article was published in 2009 and draws upon research which focuses on the period 1991 to 2005, and so perceptions may have changed since then.

Summary

This chapter has guided you in the selection of credible, relevant sources, and suggested ways in which you can engage critically with the literature. It has demonstrated how critical engagement with the literature at the reading stage is necessary in order to develop and support your own arguments when you come to writing essays or presenting work.

Sources of example texts

Brundrett, M (2013) The Importance of Teachers, Teaching and School Leaders: The 'Silver Thread' of the Reform Agenda for English Schools. Education 3-13: *International Journal of Primary, Elementary and Early Years Education*, 41(5), 459–61.

Darnell, C, Solitya, J and Walla, H (2017) Decoding the Phonics Screening Check. *British Educational Research Journal*, 43(3), 505–27.

Glazzard, J (2017) Assessing Reading Development through Systematic Synthetic Phonics. *English in Education*, 51(1), 44–57.

Hansen, A (2009) Researching 'Teachers in the News': The Portrayal of Teachers in the British National and Regional Press. Education 3-13: *International Journal of Primary, Elementary and Early Years Education*, 37(4), 335–47.

References

Beirerter, C and Sardamalia, M (1987) *The Psychology of Written Composition*. Hillsdale, NJ: Lawrence Erlbaum.

Garfield, E (2006) The History and Meaning of the Journal Impact Factor. *JAMA*, 295(1), 90–3 [online]. Available at: http://garfield.library.upenn.edu/papers/jamajif2006.pdf (accessed 5 March 2018).

Chapter 4
Critical writing

Learning outcomes

After reading this chapter you will:

- better understand what it means to write critically;

- have a better understanding of the concepts of voice, stance and argument;

- be better able to express criticality in your writing.

At the beginning of your studies, you will mainly be required to focus on describing and demonstrating your knowledge and understanding of concepts, theories and research in education. As you progress through your education degree, this knowledge and understanding will need to be increasingly underpinned by **criticality**. This chapter will further explain what criticality means, and then help you to incorporate and express criticality in your writing.

What does it mean to write critically?

As discussed in Chapter 3, Critical reading, it is important to engage critically with the literature as you research the topic of your essay. Writing critically entails making this critical engagement explicit for the reader, and using it as a platform on which to build your own argument, as you accept, reject or suspend judgement on the claims put forward in the literature.

Lecturers often cite a lack of criticality as a reason for low marks. Essays lacking in criticality are usually overly descriptive. This can mean that the writer simply reports what is in the literature, leading to a kind of 'patchwork' of other people's views. When a lecturer reads this kind of writing, they will be asking, 'But where are *you* in all this? What do *you* think now you have learned so much about the views and claims of others?' What they are looking for is your **voice**. It can be difficult to have the confidence to insert your voice in amongst the voices of respected academics and scholars, and it can take time to find and develop your own individual voice. However, it is essential if you are to be a critical writer. Criticality is essentially related to having a clear voice, having something to say, being in possession of an independent viewpoint based on an understanding of the literature and the available evidence. This viewpoint is often called your **stance**, ie your position in relation to the topic. It is not enough to state your position; you need to guide the reader through the thought processes via which you arrived at it and provide an evidence-based rationale to support it. The expression of your stance is your **argument**, the line of reasoning which is the backbone of a critical essay. You should be confident in your argument, but this does not mean being close-minded or rigid. In fact, a strong argument usually possesses significant

nuance. A nuanced argument acknowledges strengths, weaknesses and grey areas. It means sometimes qualifying your claims or recognising limitations. Last but not least, in order to make your argument clear, nuanced and persuasive, it is often necessary to use very specific **language** associated with criticality in academic writing (see for example Biber, 2006; Argent, 2017). This can involve:

- Language which specifically conveys opinion, eg 'this clearly shows', 'unfortunately', 'surprisingly'.

- Language which signals understanding of complexity in a situation, eg 'however/ although/despite/on the other hand'.

- The use of 'summary nouns' (Drummond, 2016) or 'signalling nouns' (Flowerdew, 2003), ie nouns which refer back to something previously mentioned, often signalling an element of opinion or interpretation, eg 'this decisive action', 'these so-called solutions', 'this controversial screening test'.

- Verbs and other expressions used to report, and often to interpret, what has been said or written, eg 'the consensus is'; 'Rose (2006) advocated a strong emphasis on systematic synthetic phonics'; 'there is limited evidence in this area'.

- The use of language which conveys varying degrees of certainty, especially the use of cautious language to avoid overgeneralisation or unsubstantiated claims, eg 'this appears to be a common problem'; 'there are approximately 7,000 children currently affected'; 'this suggests that teachers are…'.

CROSS REFERENCE

Academic Writing and Referencing for your Education Degree, Chapter 1, Academic writing: text, process and criticality, Writing critically

CROSS REFERENCE

Academic Writing and Referencing for your Education Degree, Chapter 2, Coherent texts and arguments, The language of criticality

Task

Identifying critical use of language

Identify the language used to convey criticality in the following text extracts.

1) It seems that teachers are under significant pressure to demonstrate that their work improves pupil outcomes, while at the same time coping with ever-increasing demands for inclusion. In order to meet these challenges, teachers must ensure that their practice is research informed.

2) Teachers may need to develop additional skills when working in urban areas. This could involve skills around supporting children whose first language is not English.

3) In conclusion, there have been a number of recent high-profile cases of racial abuse of Muslims. While these almost undoubtedly involve a minority of pupils, they clearly demonstrate the need for a renewed commitment to inclusivity and engaging pupils with British values of mutual respect for and tolerance of those with different faiths and beliefs as well as those without faith.

4) The limited benefits associated with the use of reading schemes should be weighed against the cost of providing them.

5) The authors question the effectiveness of many of the programmes that have recently been introduced to target EAL children.

Task

> ### Identifying critical essay writing
>
> Look again at the essay title from Chapter 3.
>
> **A**
>
> Outline current practice in assessing children's acquisition of phonics skills and critically evaluate the extent to which these are effective for all children.
>
> 1) In what ways does this essay title require students to engage critically with the topic and with the literature?
>
> 2) Which parts of the essay will be the least/most descriptive?
>
> 3) Read the student essay below and find examples of critical writing.
>
> 4) Can you find examples of language use which signal the student's criticality?
>
> 5) Are there any ways in which the student could have been more critical?

> ### Introduction
>
> This essay will examine different methods of assessing children's phonic knowledge, will consider the principles of effective assessment in phonics and will show how formative assessment should be used to help teachers plan the next steps in teaching. The essay will also look at diagnostic assessment, including the phonics screening check which children take in Year 1, and will examine different approaches to learning to decode and ascertain whether:
>
> a) children are being taught these in school; and
>
> b) their abilities to use phonic approaches are being assessed appropriately or, indeed, at all.
>
> Before moving on to assessment, it is important to provide some context for the current situation by describing briefly the current government-backed preferred method of teaching early reading: systematic synthetic phonics (SSP).
>
> Washtell (2010, p 44) defined SSP as 'an approach to the teaching of phonics which works by isolating the phonemes in a word. The phonemes are then blended together in sequence to decode the word'. There tends to be a systematic approach to the teaching of phonics, with letter, sound or grapheme-phoneme correspondences (GPCs) being introduced in a systematic and planned sequence. For example, in the DfES's (2007) *Letters and Sounds* programme, *s, a, t, p, i* and *n* are introduced first and are then followed by *m, d, g, o, c, k* etc. Children are taught to 'synthesise' (hence the name synthetic phonics) the sounds to form words. This is the favoured approach in the national curriculum (DfE, 2013) and it has been the subject of much debate

(see Wyse and Styles, 2007; Davis, 2013; Glazzard, 2017). SSP is the only subject knowledge element specifically required in the Teachers' Standards (DfE, 2011a), with Standard 3 including the requirement: 'if teaching early reading, demonstrate a clear understanding of systematic synthetic phonics'. Therefore, it is in the context of a strong top-down emphasis on SSP that the ensuing discussion about assessment of phonics skills will be set.

Assessing children's acquisition of phonics skills

Rose (2006) maintained that effective assessment is 'simple, rigorous and purposeful' (2006, para 61). In a survey, *Removing Barriers to Literacy*, Ofsted (2011) maintained that it was important to 'teach phonics systematically as part of the teaching of reading and ensure that pupils' progress in developing their phonic knowledge and skills is regularly assessed' (2011, p 8). Ofsted looked at schools which it identified as successful in teaching phonics and asserted that in such schools, 'the assessment of pupils' understanding of letters, sounds and words was frequent and record-keeping was meticulous' (2011, para 49).

The highly structured nature of many systematic synthetic phonics programmes lends itself to providing opportunities for regular and systematic assessment. For example, *Phonics Assessment and Tracking Guidance* (DCSF, 2009) provides assessment guidance which identifies a range of opportunities for assessment:

> This can be during the discrete daily phonics session, but will also be apparent during shared guided and independent reading and writing sessions.
>
> Writing samples provide useful evidence of children's phonic knowledge and ability to apply phonic skills, but evidence obtained through observation of children's approaches to reading unfamiliar words is of equal importance.
>
> (DCSF, 2009, p 3)

However, while there may be little controversy over the use of ongoing formative assessment to monitor pupils' progress and to help teachers determine the next steps for individual children, there has been considerable debate about the use of the national phonics screening check at the end of Year 1. For example, one study found that while the screening check does identify children who may be falling behind, it does not provide teachers with any information which could not be found through other commonly used assessments (University of Oxford, 2013). Other disadvantages included costs incurred and the tendency for schools to teach 'to the test'. Because the level of achievement required to pass the tests was set high, it was argued that this could place unnecessary pressure on young children and make parents and carers concerned.

In 2012, a survey of nearly 3000 teachers, conducted after the administration of the check but before its results, reported that 87 per cent of respondents did not agree with the statutory implementation of the check and thought that it should be discontinued (ATL/NAHT/NUT, 2012). Duff et al (2014, p 11) argued that:

> combining our observations about the integrity of the national phonics screening check data with our findings that teachers perform reliable and sensitive assessments of phonics progression, we argue in favour of using resources to continue to train and support teachers in the knowledge, assessment and teaching of early literacy skills.

Furthermore, Darnell et al (2017, p 505) questioned whether the testing of 85 grapheme-phoneme correspondences it is based on is effective. They maintained that:

> The GPCs assessed, therefore, do not reflect the full range of GPCs that it is expected will be taught within a systematic synthetic phonics approach. Furthermore, children's ability to decode real words is dependent on their vocabulary knowledge, not just their phonic skills. These results question the purpose and validity of the phonics screening check and the role of synthetic phonics for teaching early reading.

This illustrates a key point: that reading involves more than just phonics skills and that even within a phonics approach there are different strategies which readers use. These will be discussed later in this essay.

The inclusion of pseudo-words, or nonsense words, in the check has been controversial. Tal and Siegel (1996, p 224) maintain that 'the ability to decode pseudo-words indicates to what extent a child has mastered alphabetic mapping'. Gibson and England (2016) argue that in some European languages such as German, where the correspondence between graphemes and phonemes is more straightforward, there was an advantage in reading nonsense words. However, English pronunciation can vary so that a pseudo-word such as 'jound' could be pronounced to rhyme with 'found' or 'wound' (when wound refers to an injury). Gibson and England assert that such alternatives are not accounted for in the marking guidance. Another problem can be pupils' accents, and although the guidance says that accent should be taken into account, a teacher may have a preference for Received Pronunciation and mark children down if they pronounce a word with a regional accent.

The government's own website describes the screening check as follows:

Section 1
- Page 1 Four pseudo-words
- Page 2 Four pseudo-words
- Page 3 Four pseudo-words
- Page 4 Four real words
- Page 5 Four real words

Section 2
- Page 6 Four pseudo-words
- Page 7 Four pseudo-words
- Page 8 Four real words
- Page 9 Four real words
- Page 10 Four real words

All pseudo-words in the check are accompanied by a picture of an imaginary creature. This provides a context for the child (naming the type of imaginary creature) to ensure that they are not trying to match the pseudo-word to a word in their vocabulary.

(Gov.uk, 2018)

While there continues to be debate about the use of pseudo-words, schools need to prepare children for a test which includes them. During my school placement in a Year 1 class, I witnessed a teacher adopting a different approach to pseudo-words. Instead of getting the children to read nonsense words, she found lots of examples of place names which were phonically regular. She told the children that the words were the names of real places and that because they were special names they began with capital letters (capital letters are a feature of Year 1 subject knowledge). The teacher used names of towns and cities including *Tring, Diss, March, York, Hull, Leeds, Cardiff, Chard, Bridport* and *Ipswich* and was able to check children's ability to sound the phonemes and blend them to read whole words. The teacher explained to me that she needed to prepare the children for the phonics screening tests, but that she felt using place names was a much more meaningful and less confusing approach than using pseudo or nonsense words.

The effectiveness of assessment procedures for children of different abilities

We now turn to the issue of the effectiveness of assessment procedures for children of different abilities, with different learning needs and different approaches to learning to read. It is particularly interesting to note the conclusions of Glazzard in an article published in 2017, given that he is the co-author of a best-selling book on SSP:

> Different types of teaching and more comprehensive assessment batteries need to be developed to address different stages of development in reading. Given the inconclusive evidence in relation to synthetic phonics, an assessment tool which only assesses children's skills in this aspect of phonics, such as the phonics screening check, is not fit for purpose.
>
> (Glazzard, 2017, pp 52–3)

Even within their book on teaching SSP, Glazzard and Stokoe (2017) caution that the research underpinning the introduction of SSP, most notably the Clackmannanshire studies (Watson and Johnston, 1998; Johnston and Watson, 2005), were questionable in their methodology and findings. Glazzard and Stokoe go on to assert that analytic phonics has an 'important role to play in learning to read' (p 60), since English includes many rimes (for example –ight, –ing, –ack) which appear in several words which can be learned together.

Davis (2012) draws attention to another aspect of reading which may challenge those whose learning focuses heavily on sound-symbol correspondences at the expense of context: heteronyms. Davis points out that many words in English can be pronounced in different ways and that it is only when we see them in a sentence that we can be sure that our pronunciation is correct. He cites words including *tear, wind, rowing, leading, bass* and *minute* as examples.

However, in 2011, the government announced that it would provide matched funding for schools to purchase approved programmes for the teaching of systematic synthetic phonics and stated that these programmes must

> be designed for the teaching of discrete, daily sessions progressing from simple to more complex phonic knowledge and skills and covering the major grapheme/phoneme correspondences; demonstrate that phonemes should be blended, in order, from left to right, 'all through the word' for reading; ensure that as pupils move through the early stages of acquiring phonics, they are invited to practise by reading texts which are entirely decodable for them, so that they experience success and learn to rely on phonemic strategies.
>
> (DfE, 2011b)

It appears that phonics skills are understood by the government to equate to SSP, but there are other valid approaches which have been side-lined, even if they represent what most readers actually do, ie analytic, whole word and whole language approaches. In the next section, we will look at two other approaches to reading which, it will be argued, are deployed by readers to enable them to decode and comprehend text.

Analytical phonics

Analytical phonics involves a 'problem-solving' approach, as it encourages children to make links between patterns of sound found in words. For example, we know how to pronounce the word *light* so we can use our knowledge of the group of letters –*ight* to read an unfamiliar word like *dright*. Children learn to apply what they have learnt about the sounds in one word to other similar words. This might be termed analogy phonics; Brooks, (2003, p 11) describes analytic phonics as a method 'in which the phonemes associated with particular graphemes are not pronounced in isolation. Children identify (analyse) the common phoneme in a set of words in which each word contains the phonemes under study'. This approach is currently out of favour, but it would seem to be a strategy which real readers use all the time. For example, when we see an unfamiliar place name on a road sign, we may, if it is short, sound each grapheme with a corresponding phoneme to read the word, but for most words we probably make analogies with words and place names we already know in order to help us to read, for example Liverpool and Ullapool, Manchester and Dorchester.

The whole-word approach

This approach is often called the 'look and say' approach. Children are introduced to whole words through flash cards, often with accompanying pictures to link the word to its meaning. Children are taught to look carefully at words, noting their shapes and patterns, and to say the whole word. Accompanying reading schemes have incrementally more challenging vocabulary and the idea is that children will be able to read more advanced texts as their sight reading vocabulary increases. Some of these schemes also include attention to phonics, but many do not. Although, as advanced readers, we probably make considerable use of our sight vocabulary, we also need some phonic knowledge at a synthetic or analytic level when we meet an unfamiliar word.

It seems clear that while analytic and whole-word approaches may not be taught or tested in Key Stage 1 in English schools, these are strategies which real readers use.

Conclusion

This essay set out to outline current practice in assessing children's acquisition of phonics skills and to critically evaluate the extent to which these are effective for all children. It has been found that while teachers' ongoing assessment is central to successful teaching and learning, the phonics screening check has assumed a significant role in determining how teachers teach and children learn. The screening check has forced teachers who wish to see their pupils succeed to teach children to read pseudo words at a time when they are just getting to grips with real words and are beginning to enjoy reading for meaning. The screening check tests a narrow aspect of reading and does not take into account that real readers seek meaning and deploy other strategies besides breaking words into individual graphemes and sounding them out. I therefore concur with Glazzard's (2017, p 53) view that it is in fact, 'not fit for purpose'.

References

ATL/NAHT/NUT (2012) Teachers' and Head Teachers' Views of the Year One Phonics Screening Check [online]. Available at: www.teachers.org.uk/phonics (accessed 5 January 2019).

Brooks, G (2003) *Sound Sense: The Phonics Element of the NLS: A Report to the DfES*. London: DfES.

Darnell, C A, Solity, J E and Wall, H (2017) Decoding the Phonics Screening Check. *British Educational Research Journal*, 43(3), 505–27.

Davis, A (2012) A Monstrous Regimen of Synthetic Phonics: Fantasies of Research-Based Teaching 'Methods' Versus Real Teaching. *Journal of Philosophy of Education*, 46(4), 560–73.

Davis, A (2013) To Read or Not to Read: Decoding Synthetic Phonics. *Impact: Philosophical Perspectives on Education Policy*, 20, 1–38.

Department for Education (DfE) (2011a) *Teachers' Standards in England from September 2012*. London: DfE.

Department for Education (DfE) (2011b) Criteria for Assuring High-Quality Phonic Work [online]. Available at: www.education.gov.uk/schools/teachingandlearning/pedagogy/phonics/a0010240/criteriafor-assuring-high-quality-phonic-work (accessed 9 February 2019).

Department for Education (DfE) (2013) *The National Curriculum*. London: DfE.

Department for Children, Schools and Families (DCSF) (2009) *Phonics: Assessment and Tracking Guidance*. London: DCSF.

Department for Education and Skills (DfES) (2007) *Letters and Sounds*. Norwich: DCSF.

Duff, F, Mengoli, S, Bailey, A and Snowling, M (2014) Validity and Sensitivity of the Phonics Screening Check: Implications for Practice. *Journal of Research in Reading*, 38(2), 1–15.

Gibson, H and England, J (2016) The Inclusion of Pseudowords within the Year One Phonics Screening Check in English Primary Schools. *Cambridge Journal of Education*, 46(4), 491–507.

Glazzard, J (2017) Assessing Reading Development through Systematic Synthetic Phonics. *English in Education*, 51(1), 44–57.

Glazzard, J and Stokoe, J (2017) *Teaching Systematic Synthetic Phonics and Early English* (2nd ed). Northwich: Critical Publishing.

Gov.uk (2018) [online]. Available at: www.gov.uk/government/publications/phonics-screening-check-sample-materials-and-training-video/phonics-screening-check-structure-and-content-of-the-check (accessed 6 February 2019).

Johnston, R and Watson, J (2005) *The Effects of Synthetic Phonics Teaching on Reading and Spelling Attainment: A Seven Year Longitudinal Study*. Edinburgh: Scottish Executive.

Ofsted (2011) *Removing Barriers to Literacy*. Manchester: Ofsted [online]. Available at: http:/dera.ioe.ac.uk/2152/1/Removing%20barriers%20to%20literacy.pdf (accessed 9 February 2019).

Rose, J (2006) *Independent Review of the Teaching of Early Reading, Final Report, March 2006* (The Rose Review – Ref: 0201-2006DOC-EN). Nottingham: DfES Publications.

Tal, N F and Siegel, L S (1996) Pseudoword Reading Errors of Poor, Dyslexic, and Normally Achieving Readers on Multisyllable Pseudowords. *Applied Psycholinguists*, 17(2), 215–32.

University of Oxford (2013) *First Study of Government's Phonics Check Finds it is a Valid but Unnecessary Test* [online]. Available at: www.psy.ox.ac.uk/news/first-study-of-government2019s-phonics-check-finds-it-is-a-valid-but-unnecessary-test+&cd=1&hl=en&ct=clnk&gl=uk (accessed 22 December 2018).

Watson, J E and Johnston, R S (1998) Accelerating Reading Attainment: The Effectiveness of Synthetic Phonics. *Interchange*, 57. Edinburgh: SEED.

Washtell, A (2010) Getting to Grips with Phonics. In Graham, J and Kelly, A (eds) *Reading under Control: Teaching Reading in the Primary School*. Oxon: Routledge.

Wyse, D and Styles, M (2007) Synthetic Phonics and the Teaching of Reading: The Debate Surrounding England's 'Rose Report'. *Literacy*, 41(1), 35–42.

Task

Identifying opportunities for criticality

Look again at the essay title from Chapter 3.

B

Critically evaluate public and political perceptions of the role of the teacher and perceptions of the impact teachers can have upon pupils' learning.

 1) Look at the student's essay outline and notes below and decide which parts will be the most/least descriptive/analytical and evaluative.

2) Identify opportunities for critical engagement with the topic and the literature.

Introduction

- Define public and political perceptions.

- Give brief contextual background: changes to schools over last 30 or so years: national curriculum, literacy and numeracy strategies, Ofsted, local management, academies, free schools, governance, industrial action, workload.

- Identify key government interventions.

- Explain how I intend to answer the question.

Main section

- How has the role of the teacher changed?

- Give examples of media coverage of teachers.

- Use Hansen article and research to illustrate changes over time; cite Everton et al on public perceptions of teachers.

- Use case study of three teachers who have been teaching for over 30 years to exemplify (note the limitations of such a small-scale study). Do my findings accord with their experience?

Summary/Conclusion

- Bring ideas together and summarise findings.

- Draw conclusions about changing perceptions of teachers.

- Discuss implications for the future of school education.

Summary

This chapter has explored what it means to write critically. It has discussed the place of voice, stance and argument in critical writing, and highlighted the importance of careful language use. It has demonstrated the characteristics of critical writing with reference to examples of typical student writing. It has thus provided tools which will help you to write critically in your essays.

References

Argent, S (2017) The Language of Critical Thinking [online]. Available at: www.baleap. org/event/eap-northcritical-thinking (accessed 5 March 2018).

Biber, D (2006) Stance in Spoken and Written University Registers. *Journal of English for Academic Purposes*, 5(2), 97–116.

Drummond, A (2016) An Investigation of Noun Frequencies in Cohesive Nominal Groups. *Journal of Second Language Teaching and Research*, 5(1), 62–88.

Flowerdew, J (2003) Signalling Nouns in Discourse. *English for Specific Purposes*, 22(4), 329–46.

Appendix 1
Academic levels at university

UNDERGRADUATE STUDY			
England, Wales, Northern Ireland	Scotland	Award	Notes
Level 4	Level 7	Certificate of Higher Education (CertHE)	
Level 5	Level 8	Diploma of Higher Education (DipHE) Foundation Degree (FdD)	
Level 6	Level 9	Ordinary Bachelor Degree eg BA Education	Minimum academic qualification for teachers in England, Wales and Northern Ireland
	Level 10	Bachelor Degree with Honours eg BA (Hons) Education, BEd (Hons)	Usual academic qualification for teachers in England, Wales and Northern Ireland
POSTGRADUATE STUDY			
Level 7	Level 11	Masters Degree, eg MSc, MA, MPhil Postgraduate Certificate or Diploma (PGCert; PGDip)	Useful qualification for those wishing to advance their career
Level 8	Level 12	Research Doctorate (PhD) Professional Doctorate	Useful qualification for advancing careers, especially for working in teacher education in universities

Appendix 2
Verb forms in English

As you write, your choice of verb form will provide important information for your reader as regards when something occurred, how this occurrence is or should be viewed, and how it relates to the current time and context.

Verbs in English possess three important elements:

- **tense** (past, present, future), indicating the time or period in which something occurred;
- **aspect** (simple, continuous, perfect), indicating how the occurrence is perceived;
- **voice** (active, passive), indicating whether the focus is on the action itself or on the agency of the action (ie the person or thing doing it).

Some examples of common uses in academic writing are presented below with explanations as regards usage.

1) Present simple and continuous

The present simple is used for facts:

> Most children **feel** anxiety at some point in their lives.
> The lunch boxes **are found** in the trolleys in the corridor.

In the first sentence, it is important that we know who feels something (children), so the active voice is used. In the second sentence, it is the location which is important, not a hypothetical 'finder', hence the passive voice. The passive is common in academic writing as it allows for an impersonal style, eg 'it is believed that' rather than 'people believe'.

The present continuous describes current actions or developments:

> I **am** currently **working** in a primary school.
> Attitudes towards young LGBT people **are changing**.

2) Past simple

The past simple can be used to narrate a series of events, and so is commonly used in the descriptive sections of reflective writing:

> I **started** my placement in June.
> The child **was admitted** to a primary school.

In the first sentence, the agent of the action (I) is important, reflected in the active verb form; in the second sentence, the exact identity of the agent (the person who admitted the child) is unknown or unimportant in this case, hence the passive verb form.

The past simple is also common when reporting on particular studies or methodologies when reviewing the literature, with the passive voice frequently occurring in the latter, as agency can be presumed:

Joliffe et al (2015) **found** that reading improved over time.
The pupils **were monitored** over a period of six months.

3) Present perfect

The present perfect relates an action or a state to the present in some way.

There **has been** a great deal of research in this area.

(This has happened over a time period stretching to the present time.)

The government **has committed** itself to improved funding of education.

(This happened some time before the present moment, but we are not concerned with the precise time – we are more concerned with *what* has happened, not *when*.)

4) Future verb forms

There is no single future verb form in English; many forms are used to refer to the future, depending on how the action is viewed.

This policy **will have** an adverse effect on the recruitment of teachers.

(a prediction)

I'**m meeting** my mentor next week.

(an arrangement)

I'**m going to** visit several inner city schools to find out more about working with children for whom English is a second or third language.

(an intention)

These verb forms are very common in the concluding sections of reflections, when considering planned actions and future practice.

Further reading

Bottomley, J (2014) *Academic writing for international students of science.* London: Routledge.

Caplan, N (2012) *Grammar choices for graduate and professional writers.* Ann Arbour, MI: University of Michigan Press.

Answer key

Chapter 2, Reflective practice

Critically evaluating reflective frameworks

Task, Comparing and contrasting reflective frameworks (Page 25)

BROOKFIELD'S FOUR LENSES	GIBBS' REFLECTIVE CYCLE	JOHNS' MODEL
Description and evaluation Self – personal experiences The students' eyes Colleagues' perceptions	Description – What happened? Feelings – What were you thinking and feeling?	Description of the experience Reflection
	Evaluation What was good or bad about the experience? What sense can you make of the situation? What else could you have done?	Evaluation Influencing factors Could I have dealt with it better?
Learning Academic research	Learning If it arose again, what would you do?	Learning – What will change? How has this experience changed my way of knowing?

The language of reflection

Task, Identifying useful words and phrases (Pages 35–36)

1) Reflection on current knowledge and attitudes – E

2) Describing feelings – C

3) Highlighting important points – A

4) Signalling how the situation or event has challenged previous thinking – B

5) Impact on practice – D

Chapter 4, Critical writing

What does it mean to write critically?

Task, Identifying critical use of language (Page 56)

1) **It seems that** teachers are under **significant** pressure to demonstrate that their work improves pupil outcomes, while at the same time coping with ever-increasing demands for inclusion. In order to meet **these challenges**, teachers **must** ensure that their practice is research informed.

2) Teachers **may** need to develop additional skills when working in urban areas. This **could** involve skills around supporting children whose first language is not English.

3) **In conclusion**, there have been a number of recent high-profile cases of racial abuse of Muslims. While these **almost undoubtedly** involve a minority of pupils, they **clearly demonstrate** the need for a renewed commitment to inclusivity and engaging pupils with British values of mutual respect for and tolerance of those with different faiths and beliefs as well as for those without faith.

4) The **limited benefits** associated with the use of reading schemes **should** be weighed against the cost of providing them.

5) The authors **question** the effectiveness of many of the programmes that have recently been introduced to target EAL children.

Task, Identifying critical essay writing (Pages 56–64)

1) and 2) see below

This part of the essay title allows you to be descriptive. (Note the word 'outline'.)

Outline current practice in assessing children's acquisition of phonics skills and critically evaluate the extent to which these are effective for all children.

This part of the essay title demands that you are critical ('critically evaluate'). You cannot merely be descriptive here.

3) and 4) see below

Introduction

This essay will examine different methods of assessing children's phonic knowledge and will consider the principles of effective assessment in phonics and will show how formative assessment should be used to help teachers plan the next steps in teaching. The essay will also look at diagnostic assessment, including the phonics screening check which children take in Year 1, and will examine different approaches to learning to decode and ascertain whether:

a) children are being taught these in school; and

b) their abilities in these approaches are being assessed appropriately or, indeed, at all.

States key questions which will be explored.

Signpost for reader.

Before moving on to assessment, it is important to provide some context for the current situation by describing briefly the current government-backed preferred method of teaching early reading: systematic synthetic phonics (SSP).

Provides context.

Washtell (2010, p 44) defined SSP as 'an approach to the teaching of phonics which works by isolating the phonemes in a word. The phonemes are then blended together in sequence to decode the word'. There tends to be a systematic approach to the teaching of phonics, with letter, sound or grapheme-phoneme correspondences (GPCs) being introduced in a systematic and planned sequence. For example, in the DfES's (2007) *Letters and Sounds* programme, *s, a, t, p, i* and *n* are introduced first and are then followed by *m, d, g, o, c, k* etc. Children are taught to 'synthesise' (hence the name synthetic phonics) the sounds to form words. This is the favoured approach in the national curriculum (DfE, 2013) and it has been the subject of much debate (see Wyse and Styles, 2007; Davis, 2013; Glazzard, 2017). SSP is the only subject knowledge element specifically required in the Teachers' Standards (DfE, 2011a), with Standard 3 including the requirement: 'if teaching early reading, demonstrate a clear understanding of systematic synthetic phonics'. Therefore, it is in the context of a strong top-down emphasis on SSP that the ensuing discussion about assessment of phonics skills will be set.

Draws attention to the fact that this is a controversial topic.

Reminds reader of context and sets agenda for next sections.

Assessing children's acquisition of phonics skills

Rose (2006) maintained that effective assessment is 'simple, rigorous and purposeful' (2006, para 61). In a survey, *Removing Barriers to Literacy*, Ofsted (2011) maintained that it was important to 'teach phonics systematically as part of the teaching of reading and ensure that pupils' progress in developing their phonic knowledge and skills is regularly assessed' (2011, p 8). Ofsted looked at schools which it identified as successful in teaching phonics and asserted that in such schools, 'the assessment of pupils' understanding of letters, sounds and words was frequent and record-keeping was meticulous' (2011, para 49).

The highly structured nature of many systematic synthetic phonics programmes lends itself to providing opportunities for regular and systematic assessment. For example, *Phonics Assessment and Tracking Guidance* (DCSF, 2009) provides assessment guidance which identifies a range of opportunities for assessment:

> This can be during the discrete daily phonics session, but will also be apparent during shared guided and independent reading and writing sessions.

> Writing samples provide useful evidence of children's phonic knowledge and ability to apply phonic skills, but evidence obtained through observation of children's approaches to reading unfamiliar words is of equal importance.

(DCSF, 2009 p 3)

However, while there may be little controversy over the use of ongoing formative assessment to monitor pupils' progress and to help teachers determine the next steps for individual children, there has been considerable debate about the use of the national phonics screening check at the end of Year 1. For example, one study found that while the screening check does identify children who may be falling behind, it does not provide teachers with any information which could not be found through other commonly used assessments (University of Oxford, 2013). Other disadvantages included costs incurred and the tendency for schools to teach 'to the test'. Because the level of achievement required to pass the tests was set high, it was argued that this could place unnecessary pressure on young children and make parents and carers concerned.

Shows that author knows there is an issue to be critically analysed.

In 2012, a survey of nearly 3000 teachers, conducted after the administration of the check but before its results, reported that 87 per cent of respondents did not agree with the statutory implementation of the check and thought that it should be discontinued (ATL/NAHT/NUT, 2012). Duff et al (2014, p 11) argued that:

> combining our observations about the integrity of the national phonics screening check data with our findings that teachers perform reliable and sensitive assessments of phonics progression, we argue in favour of using resources to continue to train and support teachers in the knowledge, assessment and teaching of early literacy skills.

Words like 'furthermore' emphasise an additional issue of importance.

Furthermore, Darnell et al (2017, p 505) questioned whether the testing of 85 grapheme-phoneme correspondences it is based on is effective. They maintained that:

> The GPCs assessed, therefore, do not reflect the full range of GPCs that it is expected will be taught within a systematic synthetic phonics approach. Furthermore, children's ability to decode real words is dependent on their vocabulary knowledge, not just their phonic skills. These results question the purpose and validity of the phonics screening check and the role of synthetic phonics for teaching early reading.

Shows an appreciation of what the research has stated.

This illustrates a key point: that reading involves more than just phonics skills and that even within a phonics approach there are different strategies which readers use. These will be discussed later in this essay.

Makes it clear that the key points will be discussed.

Paragraph opener which indicates that this issue will be discussed further.

The inclusion of pseudo-words, or nonsense words, in the check has been controversial. Tal and Siegel (1996, p 224) maintain that 'the ability to decode pseudo-words indicates to what extent a child has mastered alphabetic mapping'. Gibson and England (2016) argue that in some European languages such as German, where the correspondence between graphemes and phonemes is more straightforward, there was an advantage in reading nonsense words. However, English pronunciation can vary so that a pseudo-word such as 'jound' could be pronounced to rhyme with 'found' or 'wound' (when wound refers to an injury). Gibson and England assert that such alternatives are not accounted for in the marking guidance. Another problem can be pupils' accents, and although the guidance says that accent should be taken into account, a teacher may have a preference for Received Pronunciation and mark children down if they pronounce a word with a regional accent.

Here the student identifies valuable points about accent and use of pseudo-words but doesn't build on them in terms of what it means for the current situation. Also, no ways forward are suggested. The problem is just stated instead of being interrogated and solutions offered.

The government's own website describes the screening check as follows:

Section 1

- Page 1 Four pseudo-words
- Page 2 Four pseudo-words
- Page 3 Four pseudo-words
- Page 4 Four real words
- Page 5 Four real words

Section 2

- Page 6 Four pseudo-words
- Page 7 Four pseudo-words
- Page 8 Four real words
- Page 9 Four real words
- Page 10 Four real words

All pseudo-words in the check are accompanied by a picture of an imaginary creature. This provides a context for the child (naming the type of imaginary creature) to ensure that they are not trying to match the pseudo-word to a word in their vocabulary.

(Gov.uk, 2018)

Sets theoretical debate within the reality of school life.

While there continues to be debate about the use of pseudo-words, schools need to prepare children for a test which includes them. During my school placement in a Year 1 class, I witnessed a teacher adopting a different

Draws upon own experience to add another perspective and to show that the author understands the practical implications of teaching pseudo words.

approach to pseudo-words. Instead of getting the children to read nonsense words, she found lots of examples of place names which were phonically regular. She told the children that the words were the names of real places and that because they were special names they began with capital letters (capital letters are a feature of Year 1 subject knowledge). The teacher used names of towns and cities including *Tring, Diss, March, York, Hull, Leeds, Cardiff, Chard, Bridport* and *Ipswich* and was able to check children's ability to sound the phonemes and blend them to read whole words. The teacher explained to me that she needed to prepare the children for the phonics screening tests, but that she felt using place names was a much more meaningful and less confusing approach than using pseudo or nonsense words.

> This paragraph lacks any research evidence to back up the teacher's practice. The idea runs the risk of being treated as unsubstantiated claims.

The effectiveness of assessment procedures for children of different abilities

> Signpost for the reader.

We now turn to the issue of the effectiveness of assessment procedures for children of different abilities, with different learning needs and different approaches to learning to read. It is particularly interesting to note the conclusions of Glazzard in an article published in 2017, given that he is the co-author of a best-selling book on SSP:

> Indicates critical interpretation.

> Different types of teaching and more comprehensive assessment batteries need to be developed to address different stages of development in reading. Given the inconclusive evidence in relation to synthetic phonics, an assessment tool which only assesses children's skills in this aspect of phonics, such as the phonics screening check, is not fit for purpose.

> (Glazzard, 2017, pp 52–3)

> Critical interpretation which emphasises that the author has both engaged with and interpreted two texts by the same authors.

Even within their book on teaching SSP, Glazzard and Stokoe (2017) caution that the research underpinning the introduction of SSP, most notably the Clackmannanshire studies (Watson and Johnston, 1998; Johnston and Watson, 2005), were questionable in their methodology and findings. Glazzard and Stokoe go on to assert that analytic phonics has an 'important role to play in learning to read' (p 60), since English includes many rimes (for example *–ight, –ing, –ack*) which appear in several words which can be learned together.

Davis (2012) draws attention to another aspect of reading which may challenge those whose learning focuses heavily on sound-symbol correspondences at the expense of context:

heteronyms. Davis points out that many words in English can be pronounced in different ways and that it is only when we see them in a sentence that we can be sure that our pronunciation is correct. He cites words including *tear, wind, rowing, leading, bass* and *minute* as examples.

The argument is meaningful but it is not supported by bringing in other research evidence about the same issue. Criticality entails a clear and confident refusal to accept the conclusions of other writers without evaluating the arguments and evidence that they provide.

Indicates another perspective.

However, in 2011, the government announced that it would provide matched funding for schools to purchase approved programmes for the teaching of systematic synthetic phonics and stated that these programmes must

> be designed for the teaching of discrete, daily sessions progressing from simple to more complex phonic knowledge and skills and covering the major grapheme/phoneme correspondences; demonstrate that phonemes should be blended, in order, from left to right, 'all through the word' for reading; ensure that as pupils move through the early stages of acquiring phonics, they are invited to practise by reading texts which are entirely decodable for them, so that they experience success and learn to rely on phonemic strategies.

(DfE, 2011b)

Shows interpretation and criticality. Note the slightly tentative phrasing: it appears that...

It appears that phonics skills are understood by the government to equate to SSP, but there are other valid approaches which have been side-lined, even if they represent what most readers actually do, ie analytic, whole word and whole language approaches. In the next section, we will look at two other approaches to reading which, it will be argued, are deployed by readers to enable them to decode and comprehend text.

Analytical phonics

Analytical phonics involves a 'problem-solving' approach, as it encourages children to make links between patterns of sound found in words. For example, we know how to pronounce the word light so we can use our knowledge of the group of letters –ight to read an unfamiliar word like *dright.* Children learn to apply what they have learnt about the sounds in one word to other similar words. This might be termed analogy phonics; Brooks, (2003, p 11) describes analytic phonics as a method 'in which the phonemes associated with particular graphemes are not pronounced in isolation. Children identify (analyse) the common phoneme in a set of words in which each word contains the phonemes under study'. This approach is currently out of favour, but it would seem to be a strategy which real readers use all the time. For example, when we see

Paragraph opener sets the agenda for the paragraph to provide more detail.

Needs research evidence to support this point.

Tentative statement shows critical interpretation.

an unfamiliar place name on a road sign, we may, if it is short, sound each grapheme with a corresponding phoneme to read the word, but for most words we probably make analogies with words and place names we already know in order to help us to read, for example Liverpool and Ullapool, Manchester and Dorchester.

The whole-word approach

This approach is often called the 'look and say' approach. Children are introduced to whole words through flash cards, often with accompanying pictures to link the word to its meaning. Children are taught to look carefully at words, noting their shapes and patterns, and to say the whole word. Accompanying reading schemes have incrementally more challenging vocabulary and the idea is that children will be able to read more advanced texts as their sight reading vocabulary increases. Some of these schemes also include attention to phonics, but many do not. Although, as advanced readers, we probably make considerable use of our sight vocabulary, we also need some phonic knowledge at a synthetic or analytic level when we meet an unfamiliar word.

> Paragraph opener sets the agenda for the paragraph to provide more detail.

It seems clear that while analytic and whole-word approaches may not be taught or tested in Key Stage 1 in English schools, these are strategies which real readers use.

> Phrases such as this show the author can draw conclusions.

Conclusion

This essay set out to outline current practice in assessing children's acquisition of phonics skills and to critically evaluate the extent to which these are effective for all children. It has been found that while teachers' ongoing assessment is central to successful teaching and learning, the phonics screening check has assumed a significant role in determining how teachers teach and children learn. The screening check has forced teachers who wish to see their pupils succeed to teach children to read pseudo words at a time when they are just getting to grips with real words and are beginning to enjoy reading for meaning. The screening check tests a narrow aspect of reading and does not take into account that real readers seek meaning and deploy other strategies besides breaking words into individual graphemes and sounding them out. I therefore concur with Glazzard's (2017, p 53) view that it is in fact, 'not fit for purpose'.

> Strong verb use shows author's opinion.

> Key concluding comment.

> Draws a strong conclusion, but there hasn't been enough engagement with other points of view to come to this conclusion.

References

ATL/NAHT/NUT (2012) Teachers' and Head Teachers' Views of the Year One Phonics Screening Check [online]. Available at: www.teachers.org.uk/phonics (accessed 5 January 2019).

Brooks, G (2003) *Sound Sense: The Phonics Element of the NLS: A Report to the DfES*. London: DfES.

Darnell, C A, Solity, J E and Wall, H (2017) Decoding the Phonics Screening Check. *British Educational Research Journal,* 43(3), 505–27.

Davis, A (2012) A Monstrous Regimen of Synthetic Phonics: Fantasies of Research-Based Teaching 'Methods' Versus Real Teaching. *Journal of Philosophy of Education,* 46(4), 560–73.

Davis, A (2013) To Read or Not to Read: Decoding Synthetic Phonics. *Impact: Philosophical Perspectives on Education Policy,* 20, 1–38.

Department for Education (DfE) (2011a) *Teachers' Standards in England from September 2012*. London: DfE.

Department for Education (DfE) (2011b) Criteria for Assuring High-Quality Phonic Work [online]. Available at: www.education.gov.uk/schools/teachingandlearning/pedagogy/phonics/a0010240/criteriafor-assuring-high-quality-phonic-work (accessed 9 February 2019).

Department for Education (DfE) (2013) *The National Curriculum*. London: DfE.

Department for Children, Schools and Families (DCSF) (2009) *Phonics: Assessment and Tracking Guidance*. London: DCSF.

Department for Education and Skills (DfES) (2007) *Letters and Sounds*. Norwich: DCSF.

Duff, F, Mengoli, S, Bailey, A and Snowling, M (2014) Validity and Sensitivity of the Phonics Screening Check: Implications for Practice. *Journals of Research in Reading,* 38(2), 1–15.

Gibson, H and England, J (2016) The Inclusion of Pseudowords within the Year One Phonics Screening Check in English Primary Schools. *Cambridge Journal of Education,* 46(4), 491–507.

Glazzard, J (2017) Assessing Reading Development through Systematic Synthetic Phonics. *English in Education,* 51(1), 44–57.

Glazzard, J and Stokoe, J (2017) *Teaching Systematic Synthetic Phonics and Early English* (2nd ed). Northwich: Critical Publishing.

Gov.uk (2018) [online]. Available at: www.gov.uk/government/publications/phonics-screening-check-sample-materials-and-training-video/phonics-screening-check-structure-and-content-of-the-check (accessed 6 February 2019).

Johnston, R and Watson, J (2005) *The Effects of Synthetic Phonics Teaching on Reading and Spelling Attainment: A Seven Year Longitudinal Study*. Edinburgh: Scottish Executive.

Ofsted (2011) *Removing Barriers to Literacy*. Manchester: Ofsted [online]. Available at: http:/dera.ioe.ac.uk/2152/1/Removing%20barriers%20to%20literacy.pdf (accessed 9 February 2019).

Rose, J (2006) *Independent Review of the Teaching of Early Reading, Final Report, March 2006* (The Rose Review – Ref: 0201-2006DOC-EN). Nottingham: DfES Publications.

Tal, N F and Siegel, L S (1996) Pseudoword Reading Errors of Poor, Dyslexic, and Normally Achieving Readers on Multisyllable Pseudowords. *Applied Psycholinguists*, 17(2), 215–32.

University of Oxford (2013) First Study of Government's Phonics Check Finds it is a Valid but Unnecessary Test [online]. Available at: www.psy.ox.ac.uk/news/first-study-of-government2019s-phonics-check-finds-it-is-a-valid-but-unnecessary-test+&cd=1&hl=en&ct=clnk&gl=uk (accessed 22 December 2018).

Watson, J E and Johnston, R S (1998) Accelerating Reading Attainment: The Effectiveness of Synthetic Phonics. *Interchange*, 57. Edinburgh: SEED.

Washtell, A (2010) Getting to Grips with Phonics. In Graham, J and Kelly, A (eds) *Reading under Control: Teaching Reading in the Primary School*. Oxon: Routledge.

Wyse, D and Styles, M (2007) Synthetic Phonics and the Teaching of Reading: The Debate Surrounding England's 'Rose Report'. *Literacy*, 41(1), 35–42.

Task, Identifying opportunities for criticality (Pages 64–65)

Introduction

- Define public and political perceptions. *descriptive*
- Give brief contextual background: changes to schools over last 30 or so years: national curriculum, literacy and numeracy strategies, Ofsted, local management, academies, free schools, governance, industrial action, workload. *descriptive*
- Identify key government interventions. *critical appraisal, eg what impact have they had and how they have been implemented and interpreted; avoid being too descriptive here*
- Explain how I intend to answer question. *signpost*

Main section

- How has the role of the teacher changed? *critically determine*
- Give examples of media coverage of teachers. *descriptive but also with critical appraisal of examples*
- Use Hansen article and research to illustrate changes over time; cite Everton et al on public perceptions of teachers. *critical element*
- Use case study of three teachers who have been teaching for over 30 years to exemplify (note the limitations of such a small-scale study). Do my findings accord with their experience? *critical element*

Summary/Conclusion

- Bring ideas together and summarise findings. *descriptive*
- Draw conclusions about changing perceptions of teachers. *evaluative summary*
- Discuss implications for the future of school education. *critical element*

Index